CHAPTERS

INTRODUCTION

Prostate cancer is a family disease, not just a man's problem. Many men die of this disease because they fail to get an annual prostate examination. They do not know that the only way to prevent death from prostate cancer is to diagnose it while it is still at an early, curable stage -usually without symptoms. Having this information could save the lives of 41,000 men who die in the United States from prostate cancer each year. It is the most common malignancy in men today.

The inspiration for this book comes from my husband who was saved from prostate cancer eight years ago. I want to help save other lives by educating men and their loved ones about the prostate gland, prostate cancer, and its treatments.

After Jim's life was saved in March of 1993, Dr. Ross Cohen and I spent many hours discussing prostate cancer and ways to prevent men from dying from it. We soon realized that the answer could only come from educating the public. But first, I had to document the need for such education. I surveyed many men from all walks of life to measure their knowledge about the prostate gland and its disorders. What I found was startling. For example, most people thought that prostate cancer could not be inherited when, in reality, it is a family disease that can be passed on from either side of the family.

The next step was to determine the most effective method of teaching men and their loved ones about prostate cancer. I considered writing a short brochure or an in-depth book; producing a videotape or even organizing support groups. Based on my interviews, I found that most people would prefer a comprehensive yet easy-to-understand book.

I also found out that men wanted to know where the prostate is located and how it works. While they were most interested in prostate cancer, they also wanted to know how to distinguish this disease from other common disorders of the gland, such as benign prostatic hyperplasia, or BPH (non-cancerous enlargement of the prostate). They wanted to know how prostate cancer is treated and what treatment options were available. And they wanted to know how to cope with the side effects of treatment, such as incontinence and impotence. What they needed most was to be informed so they could work with their physician to find the best way to manage their disease. I learned that men were eager to hear from others who have been treated for prostate cancer. Knowing how to get in touch with local, regional, and national support groups was another priority.

After listening to these men and their families, I wrote the book you are about to read: "Miracle Hands". I sincerely hope this book will provide encouragement to those with, and without, prostate cancer. The testimonies of these survivors are a vital reminder that prostate cancer need not be a death sentence; that men who have the disease, if treated early, can not only survive, but also thrive.

The message of this book is very simple. The prostate gland is important. Take care of it. Get it checked annually. If cancer is found, do not despair; effective, safe treatments are available. Most important, a regular PSA test is vital to all men between the ages of forty-five and sixty-five. For all men suffering unnecessary pain because of their lack of knowledge, this book will show how to act in time to prevent further damage and more serious problems. For any man undergoing treatment, it will give confidence every step of the way. For all men, it can dispel the myths that are counter-productive in the care of common, but commonly manageable, male medical problems.

I sincerely hope you enjoy reading the inspiring, educational, and compassionate story of a truly dedicated surgeon and urologic oncologist, Dr. Ross Cohen, who, after many years in medical practice, deserves this recognition.

Nothing in life is to be feared - It is only to be understood. - Madame Curie

DEDICATION

To my loving husband and best friend, James, a prostate cancer survivor, who has given me the strength, confidence, and encouragement to take on this tremendous challenge, and who was very instrumental in my writing this book.

To the parents and wife of Dr. Ross Cohen for their patience, support, and understanding, as well as for listening to the endless conversations about prostate cancer.

To Dr. Harry Miller, chairman of Urology at George Washington University, as well as Dr. Arnold Kwart, chairman of the Urology Department at Washington Hospital Center, for their time spent enlightening me with the background and training of one of their brightest and most talented students, Dr. Ross Cohen.

To Dr. Richard Levene, assistant Medical director, Palm Beach County Hospice, for the time he spent with me understanding how important "dignity" is when someone becomes terminally ill.

To the many colleagues in several support groups who stimulated my thinking and guided me in researching and writing this book.

Many thanks to Audrey Osterlitz and Gwen Rizzo for the endless hours spent editing this book and time devoted to making it a reality.

Finally, to the memory of my father and mother, sister Sophie, brothers Stephen and Walter, as well as the father-in-law of Roy Cohen, all who have passed on. I am trying to make a difference and need their help to continue my purpose in life.

MIRACLE HANDS

A talented surgeon's up-to-date information

on prostate problems, diagnosis,

as well as treatment options.

HELEN Y. DOYLE

Published by **Mandrill**
A division of Trident Media Company
801 N Pitt Street, Suite 123
Alexandria, VA 22314 USA

PREFACE

Prostate cancer is "the" cancer of the 1990s. As more public figures have made public that they have prostate cancer, it has become a frequent news item and topic of discussion throughout the country.

Prostate cancer has touched the lives of high profile people such as golfer Arnold Palmer, Senator Bob Dole, retired General Norman Schwarzkopf, investment broker Michael Milken, actors Telly Savalas and Don Ameche as well as New York Yankees manager Joe Torre and New York Mayor Rudolph Giuliani.

But it seems that the more we hear and read, the more confused we become. Even many primary-care doctors are confused about whether prostate cancer is a significant disease and which treatment options are best.

There are numerous books on prostate disease in general, or on men's health, but usually with only a chapter or two on prostate cancer. These books often tell you what you should be aware of about prostate cancer. But prostate cancer is too important and too controversial to confine to just a few pages.

Dr. Ross Cohen has spent a great deal of time counseling, evaluating, and treating patients with prostate cancer. His first and foremost concern is answering their questions and calming their fears by educating them.

During the last several years, Dr. Cohen has compiled a list of the questions most commonly asked by his patients. He started doing this for the patients and their families to help them better understand the disease and the various treatment options. At his patients' suggestion and urging, he and I took notes and expanded the information into this book. It provides the basic information needed to make an informed decision regarding the evaluation and treatment of prostate cancer.

We have a right to understand exactly what is going on with our body, the treatment options we have and the long-term impact on the decisions we make about our care. Hopefully, this book will educate you and answer your questions about prostate cancer.

GROWING UP

Philadelphia, Pennsylvania, has long been known as the "City of Brotherly Love." This holds true for many famous people from all walks of life who were reared in this popular city and who went on to become legends. Much of history also was made in Philadelphia. Betsy Ross in Philadelphia sewed our country's flag. Also from Philadelphia, were Benjamin Franklin, who arrived in 1723 as a penniless boy and became the first secretary of the treasury, and James Madison, who became the fourth United States president. And, the most famous name in our history, George Washington, our first president, who occupied the three-story Morris Mansion in Philadelphia for all but the first year of his two terms. We also should not forget the late Princess Grace of Monaco (former actress Grace Kelly), Eddie Fisher, and the late astronaut Charles "Pete" Conrad, who was born in the affluent Main Line suburbs of Philadelphia and was the commander of Apollo 12. They have all contributed in their own way to the American way of life.

Then too, the United States Marine Corps was formed in Ton's Tavern, Philadelphia, on November 10, 1775, a year before the Declaration of Independence was signed.

Another great name from the Philadelphia area that deserves much recognition for his talents in the medical profession is Dr. Ross Cohen, a noted surgeon and urologic oncologist.

Ross Cohen was the younger of the two children born to Herbert and Sima Cohen. His older brother, Roy, is now an attorney practicing in Summit, New Jersey.

Herb and Sima Cohen both came from the Philadelphia area, he from North Philadelphia and she from West Philadelphia. When growing up, Herb's grandmother lived across the street from Sima's aunt and uncle. Herb was a frequent visitor with his parents to his grandmother's house, spending vacations and many holidays there. As kids growing up, Sima and Herb became friends and never seemed to tire of each other. Herb went on to attend Drexel University in Drexel, Pennsylvania, and became an electrical engineer, graduating with honors. Sima remained devoted over the years, and both came to know that they wanted to spend the rest of their lives together. After marriage, Herb continued to excel in his profession and after several years he became a vice president of a major electrical construction firm which specialized in electrical construction of high-rise buildings.

After Roy and Ross were born, Herb was invited to become a partner for another electrical contractor; however, this would require quite a bit of traveling. After much consideration, Herb declined since both he and Sima were very devoted to their children and he did not want to be away from home for any length of time. They were devoted and loving parents, showing no favoritism or partiality for either boy. This was reflected in the closeness between the boys as they grew up. Sima remembers well how Ross always was a shadow behind Roy in almost everything they did. As youngsters, they enjoyed most sports, participating in baseball, track, bowling, and swimming. Herb and Sima made sure they included the boys in all their activities. As a result, there was much love and respect not only towards the parents, but also between the brothers.

When Roy and Ross were around eight- or nine-years-old, their parents decided to spend the summers in Atlantic City, New Jersey, buying a boat, which they named the 4 Cs (four Cohens). Since all the family enjoyed the water, fishing especially, the boat was a welcome addition to the Cohen household. However, whenever they came in from a fishing trip and there were fish to clean, Ross was nowhere to be found. He had a direct path to the baseball field. Ross was involved in all sports, but somehow baseball was his favorite, and for a while it looked as if he were embarking on a baseball career. Somehow, Roy always knew where to find Ross. Roy was always impressed at how confident his younger brother was in whatever task he would undertake. Nothing was ever too big and he had a solution for most of the things he did. Ross was also compassionate, even as a youngster, towards his friends. A good friend of Ross', Peter Cohen (no relation) enjoyed the water, especially fishing. As a result, the Cohens invited him on fishing trips on the 4 Cs. In fact, Ross' mother referred to Peter as the other member of the family. Peter says he will never forget Ross' kindness and compassion toward people. When Peter's younger brother passed away suddenly, the first person who called and extended his condolences and help was Ross. This was never forgotten, and they continue to be the best of friends.

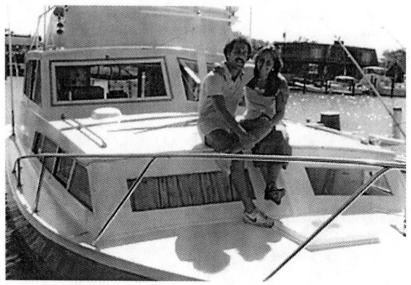

4 "C"s - Cohen's boat

When Roy and Ross were around thirteen, both boys got jobs as 'CITS" (Counselor in Training) at the Jewish Community Center in Atlantic City, New Jersey, where they spent their summers. Here they conducted themselves so well in helping underprivileged children that after two years Ross became a director of the sports camp. Not only wealthy children attended, but many poor underprivileged children as well. Ross felt that if he could make an impact on just one of these children his work at the JCC would have been invaluable.

For some reason, Ross' parents decided they wanted a change. Roy was enrolled at Rutgers University with an eye toward medicine or law when the family moved from Northeast Philadelphia to Abington, a suburb of Philadelphia. As a result, Ross transferred from the Brown School in Northeast Philadelphia to Abington High School. There he was the "new kid" trying to make new friends. He was alone now, since big brother Roy was away at college.

Amazingly, on Ross's first day in Abington High School, walking down the hall between classes, he noticed a strikingly lovely girl passing him in the opposite direction. When Ross entered his science classroom, this same lovely girl walked in and sat several seats behind him. Fortunately, Ross was wearing a football jersey with his name on the back, "COHEN." During class he would periodically turn around and look at her. Later that day in study hall, she was trying to concentrate on doing her work when Ross approached her, sat down, and started asking for help on the science homework. He found out her name was Vicki. Being very shy, Vicki was nervous and a little intimidated, but she

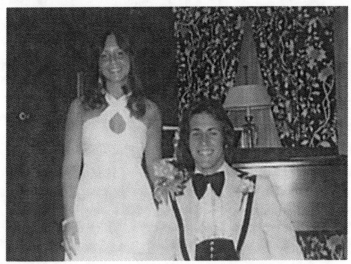

High School Prom

admitted he had the warmest smile and the sweetest personality. She was so impressed with Ross that she went home and told her mother about him. Ross, on the other hand, went home and shocked his mother by saying, "Mom, I just met the girl I am going to marry." Within a couple of days he was driving Vicki home from school and they became inseparable. One freezing winter morning, when Ross picked up Vicki to go to school, he had hot chocolate and donuts in the car. He was always so thoughtful.

Vicki graduated in June of 1975, but Ross still had his senior year to go. She left in the fall to attend the University of Maryland to study the fine arts. This was difficult for Vicki, but being apart for a year would be a good test of the strength of their relationship, so she went with confidence. Ross made the three and one-half hour drive from Abington to College Park, Maryland, on many weekends. The following fall, Ross enrolled at George Washington University in their pre-med program. Going to different schools near to one another was ideal. It allowed them to have their independent lives as well as their togetherness. After Vicki graduated in 1979, she began working as a graphic artist in Washington, DC, while Ross continued with his schooling. He started medical school at George Washington in August of 1980 and remained there, graduating with honors in May of 1984.

During Ross' third year of medical school, they became officially engaged. On Thanksgiving weekend of 1982, sitting by a fire in Ross' townhouse, sharing a bottle of champagne, Ross asked Vicki to be his wife and presented her with a beautiful ring. His parents, brother Roy, and sister-in-law had traveled from New Jersey to share the holiday with them, making that a very special and memorable weekend. Vicki's parents gave them a magnificent wedding at the Four Seasons Hotel in Washington the following June of 1983.

Ross did a two-year general surgery residency followed by a four-year urology program at George Washington University, while Vicki worked at the Watergate Complex as a computer graphics artist. In February of 1987, their first child, Adam, was born.

Ross completed his residency in 1990. Then, to his surprise, he was asked to join a urological group in Florida as a partner.

Ross has evolved over the last twenty-three years from a bright and confident teen-ager into the man he is today. It has been tremendously gratifying for his parents and family to see that all his hard work and commitment to his chosen profession has rewarded him with the ability to make a real difference in people's lives. One of the reasons Ross has succeeded as a physician is because he possesses a delicate balance of emotion and reason, compassion and objectivity, and a wonderful sense of humor with a strong sense of values. Ross is one of those rare people who seem to have an unlimited capacity to give of themselves. It is no surprise that he is such an exceptional husband and father, and why his patients have such high regard for him not only as a surgeon, but also as a human being.

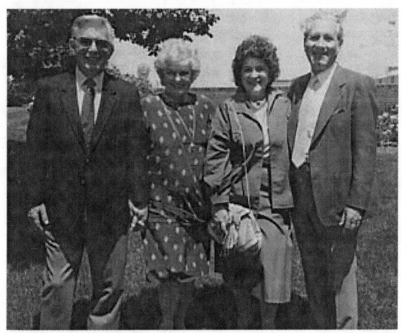

Left - Vicki's parents, Mr. and Mrs. Alspern
Right - Ross' parents, Mr. and Mrs. Cohen

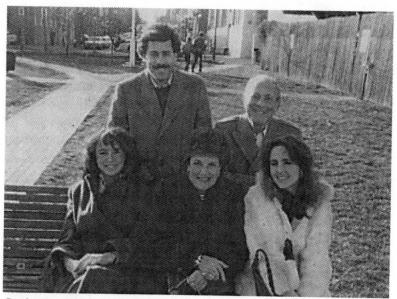

Back - Roy Cohen and father
Front - Roy's wife, Ross' mother, and Ross' wife Vicki

<u>YOUTH AND THE CALL TO MEDICINE</u>

When young and growing up, so many things go through your mind. What will I be when I grow up, will I be successful, will I have the opportunity to get a good education, and, very important, will I make my parents proud of me?

As a youngster, becoming the president of the United States is a rather far-fetched ambition. However, the thought of becoming a lawyer, doctor, pharmacist, or a corporate executive later in life is, without question, a strong possibility. Well, that is exactly what happened to Ross Cohen. When Ross was growing up, it took very little to keep him amused or occupied. In fact, as Ross' older brother Roy mentioned many times, Ross could keep himself occupied for hours on end just being constructive with his vivid imagination and natural skills. Ross admired and respected his big

19

brother Roy very much and until this day both brothers have never lost their closeness.

At the tender age of nine, Ross Cohen had the answer to the question that takes some people a lifetime to find-he knew what he wanted to become in life. And by the time he reached his eighteenth birthday, he was on his way to turning that coveted dream into a reality. Ross is what we would typically refer to as the "All American Boy." He was active in all types of sports-baseball, football, hockey, fishing, and bowling-and yet, academically, maintained excellent grades in school without trying very hard. Throughout grade school, his teachers were amazed at how curious and attentive he was, but most important, at the confidence he displayed even at an early age in any task he undertook.

Now in preparation for the medical field, he decided to take extra courses to prepare himself. He took more math, science, and advanced biology courses. But despite his heavy workload, he never gave up his love for sports or his devotion to helping underprivileged children at the Jewish Community Center.

Ross also did volunteer work in the local hospital, putting in many hours in the children's wards, reading and talking to them because he knew how important it was to see a sick child smile. From early on, it seemed that Ross was somehow destined to do well in life. And, for some reason, medicine never left his mind. By this time Vicki had enrolled at the University of Maryland, and it was no surprise when Ross applied and was accepted at George Washington University in their pre-med program.

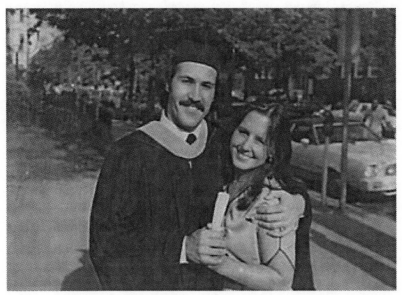

Graduation - Undergraduate School, GWU, 1980

VOCATION

In 1976 Ross enrolled in George Washington University's pre-med program. He knew this would only be the beginning of many long, tiring years before fulfilling his dream of becoming a surgeon. Ross did research on limb regeneration of adult newts and took many science courses in an effort to concentrate on applying his knowledge to humans. His original plan was to continue his involvement with children, by specializing in Pediatrics.

Ross spent his summer vacations doing volunteer work at Shore Memorial Hospital in New Jersey. Here he dealt with many major types of accidents.

Ross was deeply impressed with the realization that doctors must be men of strength and endurance far beyond that of ordinary folk. Ross himself always carried that calm, hopeful manner that gave courage and comfort to all who came under his influence. The doctors that Ross dealt with intrigued him because of their friendly interest, explaining their cases, which deepened his fascination with the subject of medicine.   It was a little incident that determined the direction he would finally take.

Ross assisted and handled many serious situations, but there was one that Ross would never forget that made a tremendous impact in his thinking about his future career. While he was on duty one evening a young girl was brought in seriously injured from a motorcycle accident. Ross was called to assist several other doctors who did everything humanly possible for her survival, but to no avail. As Ross watched her die he realized that if he could handle the trauma and stress of this situation, surgery was definitely for him.

As a result, upon completing his undergraduate school in 1980, he decided to continue medical school at George Washington University since his mind was set on surgery. During his first two years he took the basic sciences of anatomy, physiology, chemistry, botany, and pharmacology. Ross excelled in anything he did. He seemed a natural; his professors were amazed at his calm regardless of what he had to do. Basically, for the first two years, there was Medical school, the first two years cover basic science and the last two years incorporate direct patient care. After Medical school comes a residency program. Urology has two years of general surgery, followed by four years of urologic specialty training.   Here Ross was very fortunate to have the opportunity to train under the supervision of Dr. Harry Miller, chairman of Urology at George Washington University Medical Center in Washington, DC. Ross said that from the moment they met, he knew he would definitely do well under Dr. Miller's guidance. The chemistry was right between them. Ross was under Dr. Miller's supervision for approximately four years, and he excelled in everything. Consequently, Ross was invited to join the Alpha Omega Alpha Honor Society, being second highest in the class. Ross is a modest person and takes everything in stride. He simply felt it was his job to perform well.

Part of the training, under Dr. Miller's supervision, was forming a pool whereby undergraduates put their names in a hat. Doctors then picked who they thought would be best suited for a certain urology program. Since Ross and Dr. Miller were very compatible, and because of the excellent training Ross received under Dr. Miller's guidance, he now knew he wanted to specialize in urology rather than pediatrics. Dr. Miller had great faith in Ross and consequently gave him much responsibility in dealing with patients. But the responsibility was never more than he could handle. Ross reiterated often how comfortable he was working under Dr. Miller's supervision and, as a result, made many decisions on his own. He knew if he ever ran into trouble, Dr. Miller was only a phone call away. He also knew that in order to go on in his life's mission as a urologic surgeon, he would never let Dr. Miller down. Dr. Miller said that Ross seemed like a person who would definitely succeed in life. Dr. Miller went on to say that Ross was like a "sponge." You never had to squeeze him for doing additional jobs-somehow he always applied himself to everything that was needed. Ross was inquisitive and wanted to know everything that was going on and/or solutions for making things better.

Every so often, pharmaceutical companies would sponsor a medical conference whereby several doctors and their assistants or top students would participate. These meetings concerned how some of their patients reacted to various drugs or the effect of new drugs being used for cancer patients, the terminally ill, diabetic, and so on. Tapes were made at these meetings and then played later to teach the students as well as the attendees. Much knowledge was gained from these tapes, which made for a better understanding of the drugs coming to the market and their impact on patients. Dr. Miller said that usually another pharmaceutical expert or doctor would ask him questions relating to these drugs. But, when Ross came with him, he was amazed that Ross usually asked all the questions. Dr. Miller was very impressed with the manner in which Ross conducted himself. So bright, such composure, always smiling regardless of the situation, never faltering, always making you feel at ease.

Dr. Miller told me how fortunate he was to have the opportunity to have someone like Ross under his wing. As he mentioned many times over, there were many students at the medical school, but only one "Ross." He will always relish the memory of the four years Ross studied under his supervision. He always referred to Ross as the son he never had, and considered Ross part of the family. Dr. Miller also said he will never forget what a great support Vicki was for Ross. After a long day at school plus lab work, he knew Ross was completely exhausted, but after seeing Vicki, he always returned alert and ready for the next round of work.

In Dr. Miller's words, "I have nothing negative to say about Ross." He was so enthusiastic, so pleasant, had a natural mannerism with people, never stopped smiling-he just knew Ross would someday become a great doctor. Dr. Miller hoped they could keep Ross at the school to teach; but he knew in his heart that Ross was ready to make a name for himself in the real world.

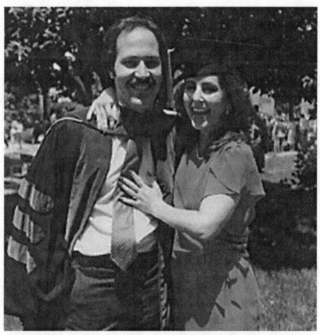

Medical School Graduation,
George Washington University, 1984

SURGICAL TRAINING

Quite a great change takes place with young interns on the house staff of a hospital. Under guidance by and permission of superiors, they can go ahead without any particular feeling of responsibility while attending to routine methods for giving practical aid to patients. When out in practice later on and assuming complete charge of cases, their methods must change.

The surgeon must learn at the outset whether he is equipped by nature to become a surgeon. Next he will learn on his own the particular sort of surgeon he is likely to become. Here and there a man of natural talent and mechanical ingenuity becomes a valuable addition to the ranks of surgery. But only doctors realize how much time, pain, imagination, mental stress, and money have gone into the making of an experienced surgeon.

A young doctor, upon graduating from medical school, swears by Hippocrates that his life will be devoted to the welfare of people without regard for his personal advantage. The practice of medicine is a game like golf or bridge, and must be played according to the rules. The ideals of medicine involve the intellect, character, and willingness to serve others. You cannot play this game for personal advantage. After completing the standard preparation in the medical profession, a young doctor usually has to learn, first, to treat well the members of the family of a patient, then the mind of the patient, and finally his or her illness.

When Ross graduated from medical school in 1984, he had the opportunity to serve his internship at many hospitals. But, since he liked and was familiar with the Washington, DC, area, he chose to remain at George Washington University. Here, Ross continued to focus on surgery. Also, his fondness for children kept him interested in pediatrics. And the thought of helping underprivileged children never left his mind. However, Ross was beginning his internship and starting the elective part of surgery rotation. Up until this point he never had any direct patient contact. But now he had the opportunity to rotate through different specialties. In other words, he would involve himself anywhere from three to six months in pediatrics, urology, general surgery, cardiology, as well as matters dealing with the ear, nose, and throat. Ross enjoyed this rotation because it gave him the opportunity to finally realize what he wanted in life.

As noted, Ross spent many hours as a volunteer talking and caring for children in the children's wards of local hospitals, hoping that his presence would bring a smile to terminally ill children. They were so attentive, so alert and more than anything, always looked forward to your return day in and day out. At this point, pediatrics still was for him. Then he had the opportunity to serve a rotation with both Dr. Harry Miller, chairman of Urology at George Washington University Medical Center in Washington, DC, and Dr. Arnold Kwart who was in private practice in Washington, DC, and a clinical professor at the same university.

Up until this point Ross felt his career was going to be in pediatrics. But when he signed up for his rotation in Urology, he felt slightly confused. After Dr. Miller and Dr. Kwart conducted their round robin rotation programs in urology, Ross' mind seemed to shift. He felt his personality was a good fit for Dr. Miller's urology program. Dr. Miller moreover was quite impressed with what he saw in Ross Cohen. Ross began to see the appeal of treating men, woman and children of all ages in a discipline that could yield rapid and visible results. He learned that urolgy is a very diversified field with a large office-based practice as well as a diverse surgical specialty. Within three months Ross knew that urology was definitely his field.

Ross continued his surgery rotations, working from three to six months at a time at various institutions-Children's Hospital, VA Medical Center in Washington, DC, Fairfax Hospital in Fairfax,

VA in addition to making private house calls to familiarize himself with all types of urological problems. Ross was fortunate enough to come under the wing of Dr. Arnold Kwart for the last four years of his training, along with that of Dr. Harry Miller. Since Dr. Kwart was in private practice as well as the urological clinical professor at George Washington University, this gave Ross a wonderful opportunity to gain much knowledge first-hand in dealings with patients. Dr. Kwart would bring his patients to the hospital for surgery and Ross would operate with him. Dr. Kwart was trained at John Hopkins Hospital in Baltimore, MD, and because of his extensive training, he became an extremely competent doctor. Dr. Kwart was very devoted to the residency program at George Washington and somehow instilled in all his trainees that hard work and dedication would always be rewarding. As a result, Ross was delighted to be chosen to work with Dr. Kwart in their urology program. Here Ross saw and participated in many surgeries that Dr. Kwart performed. These surgeries involved the colon, prostate, kidney, bladder, or any other urological problem that a person might have. Ross was impressed with Dr. Kwart's confidence.

Dr. Kwart was not only an excellent physician but also a great person. He knew if you were ready to deal with the real world after four years under his wing. Doctors don't live at the hospital, so they must decide whether a patient needs constant care; whether to be on call; or just routine. Ross always knew, because of his marvelous training, that it was his responsibility to do the right thing when dealing with patients.

Dr. Kwart spoke of the pleasure it was to have Ross under his wing because he handled himself so professionally, always calm and never faltering when making a decision. He also felt, like Dr. Miller, that without a doubt, someday soon Ross would become a great surgeon. He was a natural, adapted himself to everything so easily and his concern was always the patient. In fact, when Ross operated on my husband Jim eight years ago, Dr. Kwart mentioned that it was his voice whispering in Ross' ears that gave him the confidence he instilled in him earlier when training. This was a joke between them.

Jim never had any earlier problems-he was young for prostate cancer-and when Ross operated on him within one month of his illness, his malignancy had already spread to the other side of his prostate. But because of the skilled hands of Ross Cohen, Jim is here today. He needed no treatments and was able to return to his normal activities within three weeks. A miracle but, again, this reflects Ross'training under the guidance of two great doctors, Dr. Arnold Kwart and Dr. Harry Miller. He will never forget their training him to become the surgeon he is today.

DECISION TO RELOCATE

Ross continued his training under the marvelous guidance of both Dr. Kwart and Dr. Miller. He was becoming very comfortable with patients in the hospital and making house calls. He also had the opportunity to assist in major cancer surgery operations. His lifestyle was completely changing, and each day he was getting more and more involved with urological surgery operations which he relished since much more responsibility was being given to him. As noted, having made his decision to specialize in urology, Ross looked forward to involving himself with more surgery of the prostate, kidneys, bladder and colon.

After two years under Dr. Kwart's wing, Ross was doing operations on his own. Ross was calm and confident; but more importantly, had a tremendous bedside manner with these patients. As Dr. Kwart said, "They loved Ross," and many times only wanted to see Ross to speak of their problems. Ross was building a great reputation for himself in his chosen field He began to handle many difficult cancer surgery cases on his own. For some reason, urology and Ross' personality were a perfect fit, so it was no surprise that he was rapidly rising in the ranks of notable urologists at the hospital. He knew, however, he still had a way to go.

Ross was always a modest individual, so gaining all this recognition never fazed him. Instead it made him work harder. He definitely enjoyed his clinical rotations because it gave him the opportunity to become familiar with so many different situations.

In June 1990 Ross felt he was ready for the real world. After all his wonderful training and experience, it was time for him to make a decision. He had grown very fond of George Washington University and the surrounding area. Both Dr. Kwart and Dr. Miller tried to persuade Ross to stay and teach at the university, but in their hearts they knew this would not happen. They both knew Ross was ready to go out on his own and make a name for himself. Both Dr. Kwart and Dr. Miller knew without a doubt Ross soon would become a great doctor and make them both proud. So, Ross started to send out résumés for, like everyone else in the real world, he needed a job. He basically concentrated his efforts in New Jersey and Florida. He was surprised to get responses back so quickly. One that intrigued him most was a call from a doctor in Florida who then flew up to see Ross. The interview went very well and consequently Ross was invited to come to Florida and meet with colleagues of this doctor who ran a urological group. Ross flew down and met with the other doctors in this group. Basically this group was looking for someone with extensive cancer surgery experience that they needed at various hospitals with which they were affiliated. Since Ross had this extensive surgery experience and was familiar in all areas-bladder, kidney, prostate, and colon-he was hired to join this group. This made Ross very happy, because Florida was one place where he wanted to relocate to give his family the opportunity to enjoy the sunny atmosphere. And also that Vicki could be near her mother who lived in Boca Raton.

Ross had been given the opportunity to know all the newer techniques of the previously mentioned types of surgery. Today, as a result, he does all these types of operations at various hospitals. In fact, he is Chief of Urology at J.F.K. Hospital in West Palm Beach, Florida. He has created his own method of reconstructing a bladder so one does not have to wear an external appliance. Ross Cohen is what he is today simply because he is a real person-compassionate and dedicated through his creative techniques to saving more and more lives from this "silent disease," Prostate Cancer.

WHAT TO DO IF YOU ARE DIAGNOSED WITH PROSTATE CANCER

The prostate gland causes more grief for men than just about any other gland in the body. Prostate problems may eventually trouble more than half of all American males, but except in relatively rare cases, fear and popular falsehoods may be more dangerous than the disease itself. Few men know what the prostate actually is and does, how it inevitably changes with age, or how effective various treatments are likely to be. Most men do not understand the functions of a healthy prostate, the diseases that can affect the prostate, and treatment choices and possible after effects. Read on for the answer to most questions on topics such as prostate specific antigen and its uses, watchful waiting: for benign prostatic hyperplasia and treatment and options for prostate cancer, including cryoablation of the prostate for cancer, as well as new methods, both medical and surgical, for treatment of benign prostatic hyperplasia (BPH) as well as for prostate cancer.

The most frequent fear of patients is the loss of their sexual potency. Ironically, the fear itself may be the cause of some sexual dysfunction. The patient who takes time to understand his disease will usually recover his normal potency following procedures used to correct or relieve the problem. On the practical level, Dr. Cohen helps alleviate stress and embarrassment by explaining in detail the various techniques of prostate examination. Physical pain can be avoided, in most instances, by proper mental preparation.

There are three common diseases of the prostate - infection and inflammation, benign prostatic hyperplasia, and cancer.

The next few chapters will explain what the prostate looks like, and the various procedures and treatments.

The function of the prostate gland is to add vital nutrients and fluid to the sperm. The prostate is a relatively small, walnut-sized gland that sits just below the urinary bladder in the bottom of the pelvis surrounding the urethra. It is this position that leads to difficulties later in life. As the gland enlarges from normal growth or from cancer, it can cause narrowing of the urinary passage and make it increasingly difficult to urinate. When fathering children is no longer a goal, the prostate no longer serves its main purpose. However, the gland remains and, in the presence of normal male hormones, continues to grow until at some point it may cause problems.

The prostate is actually a collection of glands encased as one organ that secretes fluid. A thin capsule of compressed fibrous tissue surrounds it. Outside of the prostate is a layer of fat. Below the prostate, just a few millimeters away, is the front wall of the rectum. On each side are nerves and blood vessels. Dr. Cohen says that these nerves are very important when he explains the treatment choices for prostate cancer and the problems that can occur, and are the ones that must be preserved if the patient is to regain potency after surgery for prostate cancer.

The prostate is divided into right and left sides called lobes. The tip of the prostate farthest from the bladder is the apex. The wider portion next to the bladder is the base. The front is called anterior, and the rear the posterior. The vas deferens is the tube that leads the sperm from the testicles to the urethra and empties into the urethra inside the prostate. Fluid from adjacent glands called the seminal vesicles also drain into the prostate. These glands are next to the prostate and below the bladder. The testicles not only make the sperm, but also produce the male hormone testosterone, which is delivered directly into the bloodstream.

The bladder sits above the prostate, in the bottom of the pelvis. It serves two purposes. First, the bladder is a container or reservoir for urine, so you can build up urine and empty when you choose to, rather than when it is created. The second function is to serve as the muscle that squeezes out the urine when given the necessary messages from your brain. Urine is made in the kidneys by filtering waste products from the blood. The urine then drains down the urethra into the bladder.

The urethra is the tube that leads from the bladder through the prostate, past the urinary sphincter, and out the penis to the opening called the meatus. The urinary sphincter is a collection of circular muscle fibers just below the prostate that helps to prevent leakage of urine when you cough, move, or are physically active. Most of the control (called continence) of urine actually occurs at the bladder neck. There, all of the circular muscle fibers at the bladder neck come together like a funnel. Veins of the prostate drain blood out and up toward the heart alongside the spinal column. The lymphatics drain from the prostate to a number of small lymph nodes clustered along the wall of the pelvis on both sides. The lymphatics are the cleaning system for the body. All cells of the body are "bathed" by lymph fluid - clear, slippery fluid that sometimes oozes from scrapes or abrasions. This fluid is filtered through lymph nodes, where any impurities, germs or cancers are captured. The filtered lymph fluid then flows back into the bloodstream.

As Dr. Cohen informed my husband, the prostate in most men grows slowly and increases in size. This growth, called benign prostatic hyperplasia, or BPH, is not cancerous, but can seriously affect a man's quality of life by causing blockage to the urine flow. This can result in a number of annoying and bothersome symptoms such as frequent daytime and nighttime urinations, dribbling, and difficulty starting and stopping the urinary stream.

For years, treatment options for BPH were limited. Most men who had the problem ultimately had surgery. During the past decade, however, new breakthroughs and advances have provided a wide range of options that can often reduce the symptoms without the risks and potential side effects of surgery.

There are five basic options for treating the symptoms of an enlarged prostate:

1. Do nothing, observation alone.
2. Take alpha-blocker medication such as Hytrin, Cardura or

Flomax . These medicines relax the prostate at neck of bladder to allow easier flow and help alleviate the symptoms of BPH

3. Take Proscar or Saw Palmetto. Proscar is used to shrink the prostate and can take three-to-six months to work. It is medicine that must be taken long-term to keep the prostate reduced in size.

4. Have laser surgery, vaporization or microwave therapy. These are minimally invasive outpatient procedures used to shrink and relax the prostate. They are effective about 70% of the time.

5. Have a standard surgical resection of the prostate, called a transurethral prostatectomy (TURP). This remains the Gold Standard for the treatment of BPH. Tissue is scraped out of the prostate, much like taking the core out of an apple. This relieves the blockage and is successful 90% of the time.

You can always choose not to treat your symptoms. If you are not bothered much by blockage symptoms, it is reasonable to just watch and wait. You may find that you are doing better, staying the same or getting worse. Of course, if the symptoms do become a problem, then you should talk to your doctor about your other choices.

I remember how interesting it was to talk to two men who had the same problems in urinating. One was miserable getting up twice each night to urinate, while the other was thrilled that he was not getting up more often.

PROSTATE CANCER is a malignant growth of the glandular cells of the prostate. Normally these cells are located within the glands that produce the fluid that makes up most of the semen. But, under certain circumstances, these cells can lose their normal controls and start to grow out of control. Like all cancers, it probably starts as a tiny change in just a few cells. Over many years, perhaps even twenty or more, this tiny cluster gradually enlarges. As the cancer grows, it gains momentum, growing faster. Some may grow very rapidly and can be quite deadly. Prostate cancer is in a class of cancers, like breast cancer, that is hormone-sensitive. In the prostate, the hormone testosterone is converted into another very powerful hormone, DHT. In prostate cancer, these hormones stimulate the cancer cells uncontrolled growth.

As the cancer grows, it invades surrounding tissue. At first, it just grows into more of the prostate. But when the cancer reaches the outside capsule or shell of the prostate gland, the cancer can grow through this into the fat surrounding the prostate. Cancer can also grow into the adjacent bladder or the seminal vesicles. Prostate cancer spreads to two main areas of the body. First, to the lymph nodes that drain the prostate, and second, to the bone, mostly of the spine and ribs. Specifically, the cancer grows inside the bone marrow - the inside of the bone where active growth of new bone takes place.

Cancer cells leave the prostate in the bloodstream. As the blood leaves the prostate gland it travels through a web of veins alongside and into the spine. The blood then passes into the bones of the spinal column. Prostate cancer cells grow here because it is the first body environment the cells encounter that encourages their growth.

The exact causes of prostate cancer are not known. It may be years before we have any definitive answers. However, recent evidence suggests that prostate cancers may develop because of genetic imbalances. These imbalances may be accelerated by environmental factors such as diet, which can lead to mutations over time.

We do know that some genes in every cell in the body prevent cancer by blocking or suppressing cancerous changes in the tissue. When these preventive genes are blocked, there is nothing to keep the cancer from starting up and growing. There are also genes that lie dormant, but under yet unknown circumstances they activate and stimulate cancer cell growth.

Studies suggest that a high fat diet seems to stimulate prostate cancer. This is particularly true of red meat and dairy products. Prostate cancer is far less common in countries with a low fat diet, such as Japan and China. It has been found that when men move to countries with high fat diets, the risks of developing prostate cancer increase and may be as high as everyone in the local population within a generation or two. This seems to suggest diet is probably one of the factors that enables or perhaps even encourages the cancers to grow. A high fat diet serves to activate an otherwise dormant internal mechanism within a cell's own structure than directs the cell to grow without its usual limits and boundaries. Or it may block a proctive mechanism, so the cell can grow without its usual restrictions.

An individual can lower his risks for prostate cancer by following correct lifelong dietary practices. However, the world population is not likely to change to a high-fiber, low fat diet. Therefore, it is highly unlikely that the incidence of prostate cancer will ever be reduced by dietary changes alone.

There are various reasons why doctors and researchers know little about such an important cancer.

1. Little money has been invested in prostate cancer research; this despite a reminder that every ninety seconds a man in America is diagnosed with prostate cancer.
2. Prostate cancer takes so long to grow that short-term studies are not of much use. Long-term studies are difficult to start up and keep going.
3. The disease is different from person to person and each variant of the disease behaves differently. It is almost impossible to compare one treatment to another. Therefore, we need more intensive research to find a cure.

Although much is known about prostate cancer from clinical experience, significant studies are not being funded. Therefore, it is important to understand what early detection of this deadly disease means to men. Bear in mind that all men are at risk of developing prostate cancer at some point in their lifetime. As the population grows older, more prostate cancer is going to be detected. This is most often a disease of older men. However, young men, like my husband, can get prostate cancer as well. As modern medicine continues to keep us living longer with healthier lives, many of us will eventually be diagnosed with prostate cancer. In other words, if you live long enough, sooner or later you probably will develop prostate cancer. Whether or not the cancer will affect your quality of life or longevity is a different issue.

Every man over the age of fifty should routinely have a general medical examination, a digital rectal examination, a urine evaluation, and a PSA blood test. All of these can be done at the same time when you visit your primary care doctor. Giving the vital information regarding your past history to your doctor can be important in helping your physician decide if there is reason to be concerned. If something is not as it should be, then further evaluation may be appropriate.

THE PROSTATE

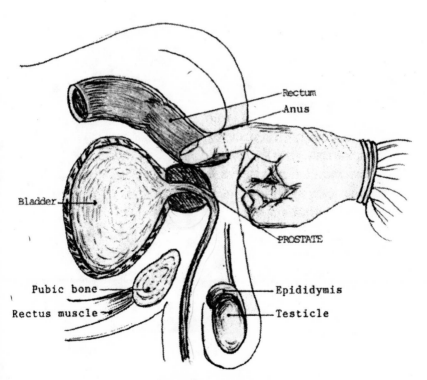

Digital rectal examination.

WHAT EVERY MAN SHOULD KNOW
ABOUT PSA

Prostate specific antigen (PSA) is a protein that is secreted by the lining of the prostate gland and is detected in the blood. Since the late 1980s, PSA has emerged as the most important tumor marker for screening, detection, staging and monitoring of men with prostate cancer. In fact, there has been a marked increase in detecting early prostate cancer and a simultaneous decline in metastatic prostate cancer between 1986 and 1996.

PSA is used along with digital rectal examination (DRE) for prostate cancer screening, and when used together, more tumors are being diagnosed at an earlier, curable stage. Currently PSA testing and DRE are recommended annually for men 50 years or older. For African American men or men of any race with a family history of prostate cancer testing should begin at the age of 40. PSA for the most part is specific for the prostate gland; however, trace amounts may be detected in some primary cancers of the lung, adrenal gland and kidneys.

The normal range for PSA levels is usually 0.0 to 4.0, although some types of PSA tests have the upper limits of normal 2.5. Results from the two types of tests are not the same; they are two different types of PSA measurements. Also, though most men with prostate cancer are diagnosed with a PSA level of less than 20, the PSA can go up into the hundreds and even into the thousands. A reading at these higher levels almost always means you have advanced prostate cancer. Usually additional tests will show the cancer may have spread to the bones or the lymph nodes.

The PSA can be elevated in men with benign prostatic hyper-trophy (BPH), prostatitis (infection of the prostate), or in men with prostate cancer. Some medications alter the PSA level. such as prostate drug Proscar. It has been shown to decrease the PSA level by 50 percent after six months of treatment.

Unlike surgery where the PSA should be 0.0, after radiation the PSA usually drops slowly down to a level ideally below 1.0. The longer it stays below 1.0, the better the long-term prognosis. However, if the PSA does not drop below 1.0, then statistically you are more likely to have a recurrence of cancer. Remember, monitoring the PSA plays an important role. As a result, if there is a question about return of the cancer, you can be followed more closely. While many men will not live long enough for the cancer to be a threat to them, others may have rapid growth and have problems almost immediately. In general, the less aggressive the cancer, the better your long-term outlook.

There have been cases where some men with infections push the PSA reading up into the 60s or higher, but with treatment it returns to normal within a few months.

There are various causes of an elevated PSA.

1. Cancer of the Prostate
2. Benign Enlargement of the Prostate Gland
3. Urinary Tract Infection/or Prostate Infection
4. Stones Within the Prostate
5. Instrumentation of the urinary tract, i.e. catheterization, prostate biopsy, cystoscopy or recent prostate surgery.

Saw palmetto, a popular prostate health food supplement, probably has minimal impact on the PSA measurement. Routine digital rectal examination has not been found to significantly elevate the PSA, but instrumentation of the prostate or urinary tract, such as with cystoscopy or prostate biopsy, can and gener-ally does increase the levels of PSA. You should, wait six to eight weeks after these manipulations to draw the PSA.

I remember Dr. Cohen being asked many times why you have to wait so long to recheck the PSA. The reason is that it takes a long time for the swelling and irritation of the tissues of the prostate gland to heal. If the PSA is checked while the swelling and irritation is still present, then the PSA will still be elevated and continue to confuse the issue. You should wait long enough for healing before the test is performed again. One of Dr. Cohen's patients, for example, was very upset that his PSA went from 3.5 to 3.9 over a six-month period. Dr. Cohen explained that this could represent a growing cancer, but most likely if the test was repeated the results would come back from 3.1 to 4.0 representing the usual day-to-day fluctuations in the level. Also, in following the progress of a man with a normal exam and a PSA around 0.8 - 1.0 every year for several years, a follow-up examination was still normal, but his PSA jumped to 2.6. After checking it was found he had no infection or other reason to explain the sudden elevation. However, subsequent evaluations showed he did have cancer of the prostate. This patient decided on surgery, which showed a surprisingly large volume of cancer, but no evidence the cancer had spread. This patient had an excellent long-term prognosis. This is because not all prostate cancers produce PSA. The PSA can rise approximately 1.0 point per year and still be normal growth of the prostate for a man.

An elevated PSA does not necessarily indicate prostate cancer, however, as a general rule the higher the PSA the more likely that a man has prostate cancer. It is estimated that a man with a PSA between 4 and 10 ng/ml has a 25 percent chance of having prostate cancer. If the PSA is 10 ng/ml, the chances increase to approximately 50 percent.

Because the PSA is not cancer-specific and varies in other prostate conditions, new ways of utilizing PSA have become popular. PSA density. Age specific PSA and PSA velocity (change in PSA over time) all attempt to account for PSA elevations. Most of the new studies have focused on the frequency of obtaining PSA measurements, fractionating PSA into the free and total PSA, and a new approach called the Prost Asure Index.

PSA DENSITY

As the prostate gland grows the PSA would likewise be expected to increase. The PSA density is calculated by dividing the PSA measured in the blood, by the size of the prostate as measured by transrectal ultrasound.

The limitation of using PSA density is that transrectal ultrasound is not a perfect measure of prostate volume. PSA density has not been shown to be much better than the standard PSA level in determining prostate cancer.

AGE SPECIFIC PSA

Age-related growth of prostate tissue has been analyzed from large numbers of patients who develop age-specific PSA.

For a man Age	Normal Range
40 - 49	0.2.5 ng/ml
50 - 59	0-3.5 ng/ml
60 - 69	0-4.5 ng/ml
70 - 79	0-6.5 ng/ml

Age-specific PSA has recently been challenged with the fear that using higher PSA cut-offs for older men may make it less likely to diagnose prostate cancer at an earlier, curable state.

PSA VELOCITY

PSA velocity monitors the PSA change over time and may be a more accurate way to evaluate the significance of a PSA blood test. A series of at least three PSA blood tests must be obtained over 1-1/2 years. If the PSA increases to greater than 0.75 ng/ml/year, then there is a suspicion that prostate cancer exists and a biopsy is indicated. It is most useful in following patients who have had a negative biopsy of the prostate but whose PSA remains elevated.

FREE AND TOTAL PSA

The evaluation of the type PSA may also be useful when considering the significance of an abnormal PSA. PSA may exist in either a free form or bound to proteins in blood.

AN ELEVATED PSA DOES NOT NECESSARILY INDICATE PROSTATE CANCER

As the percentage of free PSA decreases, the probability of having prostate cancer increases (in men with a total PSA between 4 and 10 ng/ml, those with prostate cancer tend to have a lower percentage of free PSA. For men with a percentage free PSA of 25, the risk of prostate cancer being present may be so low that prostate biopsy may be avoided.

In summary, the fact that prostate cancers usually release a form of PSA different from the PSA released by benign prostate glands provides the basis for using percent free PSA as a better indicator of prostate cancer.

THE PROSTASURE INDEX

The ProstAsure Index is a new, promising test, which at this time is in its final stages of investigation. The index takes into account several variables: the patient's age serum PSA serum, prostatic acid phosphatase. and serum creatinine kinase. A powerful computer analyzes the values from these four variables, and a ProstAsure Index value is calculated. Results show that patients with an index value greater than 0.5 are recommended to undergo prostate biopsy to determine if prostate cancer is present.

MONITORING PROSTATE CANCER

Measuring the PSA is the most effective way of monitoring patients with known prostate cancer. A rising PSA following any treatments for prostate cancer (surgery radiation or hormone therapy) provides the earliest warning of treatment failure. In patients with prostate cancer who are just being followed with watchful waiting, a rising PSA might be the first sign that treatment should be instituted. This perhaps is the single best use of the PSA as a tumor marker for patients with known prostate cancer.

It is important to remember that follow-up care will be necessary for the rest of your life after you have been treated for prostate cancer. In today's society, the PSA blood test is the best and least expensive way of making sure that the cancer has not come back after treatment. As long as the PSA level remains stable, you are doing fine. How often you need to be seen depends on your particular medical situation, the treatment you received, and how likely it is that the cancer was cured. Initially, after radiation or surgery, you will probably need to get the PSA rechecked every four months for the first year, then every six months the next four years, then once a year thereafter. The longer you go after treatment without signs of cancer recurrence, the longer you can go between PSA checks. The PSA is an excellent way of following patients after prostate cancer treatment.

If the PSA happens to go up, then it depends on how much change there has been in the PSA, to what level, and over how much time. You should remember that there is some fluctuation in

47

lab testing. Very minor changes probably do not mean anything. However, if the PSA continues to rise on three separate occasions several months apart, it means the cancer has returned. The faster the climb, the more concerned your doctor is. A rapid increase suggests that the cancer not only is back, but also is growing vigorously. But sometimes, the PSA elevation is so small and so slow, that Dr. Cohen chooses just to watch it over time. After a radical prostatectomy, the PSA level should be 0.0 to 0.2. If the PSA level starts to go up after surgery and continues to rise, this usually means that there is some recurrent prostate cancer. No one really knows when and if additional treatments should be started. Dr. Cohen says that if the PSA goes up, he would then evaluate the possibility of spread by using a CT scan. bone scan or possibly a new exam called the prostascint scan. If cancer were found in the area of the prostate bed, he would be inclined to recommend radiation to the pelvis. If the cancer is found outside of the prostate bed, or no definite site found he would likely recommend hormone therapy Unlike following surgery where the PSA should be 0.0, after radiation the PSA usually drops slowly down to a level ideally below 1.0. The longer it stays below 1.0, the better the long-term prognosis. However, if the PSA does not drop to below 1.0, then statistically you are more likely to have a recurrence of cancer. Remember, monitoring the PSA plays an important role. As a result, if there is a question about return of the cancer, you can be followed more closely. While many men will not live long enough for the cancer to kill them, others may have rapid growth and have problems almost immediately. In general, the less aggressive the cancer, the better your long-term outlook.

Cancer of the prostate can spread to the lymph nodes or bone, but it can also spread into surrounding tissues. The bone scan and CT scan show abnormalities only when recurrent cancer is large enough to produce changes in the bones or to cause fairly significant enlargement or distortion of normal tissues on CT scan. If the PSA is going up, then your doctor knows that the cancer is growing somewhere.

Dr. Cohen has stressed that measuring the PSA is the most effective way of monitoring patients with prostate cancer. A rising

PSA following any treatments for prostate cancer (surgery, radiation or hormone therapy) provides the earliest warning of treatment failure. In patients with prostate cancer who are just watchful waiting, a rising PSA might be the first sign that treatment should be instituted. This perhaps is one of the best uses of the PSA as a tumor marker for patients with known prostate cancer.

The PSA in and of itself is not a perfect diagnostic tool and, like any test, does have limitations. However, used in conjunction with sound urological judgment, it is the most important tumor marker in cancer patients today. Genetics, the study of heredity, and how one's genes and disease are related, is a promising field, whereby researchers are trying to identify which genes are responsible for development of cancer. Other questions are: why do some genes somehow allow environmental factors to stimulate prostate cancer to grow? Could this be how a high-fat diet encourages prostate cancer to grow? And, do some men have certain genes that suppress the development of prostate cancer? Can diet or the proper environment activate these protective genes? Are there certain enzymes in the body that, when blocked by a genetic change, allow cancers to grow? At present there are no answers to these questions. However, research is underway around the world to try to solve these puzzles about the origin of not only prostate cancer, but also all cancers.

TRANSRECTAL ULTRA SOUND AND BIOPSY

If you are found to have an abnormal rectal exam or elevated PSA, or both, the next step is to have a diagnosis made. Doing a transrectal ultrasound and biopsy of the prostate does this. This is where a urologist places an ultrasound probe into the rectum which allows the prostate to be examined internally with sound waves looking for abnormal areas. A biopsy is where tissue samples are taken through the ultrasound probe so that tissue can be examined to see if prostate cancer is present. Typically, six to twelve biopsies are taken in order to adequately sample the entire prostate gland.

This procedure is done in the office with some mild discomfort, but it is generally well tolerated. What you should know is that after a biopsy, you may have blood in the urine, stool or semen for up to four to six weeks. This is because the needle passes through the rectal wall and into the prostate gland, which is surrounded by many veins. Occasionally, blood can be seen in the semen for a few months after prostate biopsy. This should not cause worry. A doctor is concerned only if the bleeding is heavy and prolonged, as it can lead to difficulty urinating, requiring placement of a catheter, and, rarely, surgery under anesthesia to find the bleeding spot.

A question often asked is whether one becomes impotent after a prostate biopsy. This is very rare. However, a biopsy on a patient several years ago did have that result, but the patient had had a problem with impotence for several months following the study. It is still puzzling. However, although swelling and inflammation alongside the prostate where the nerves travel could cause a temporary problem. It would be quite rare to have enough inflammation and swelling on both sides to affect erections.

When cancer is detected in biopsied tissue, the challenge is to find out how much cancer is believed to be in the prostate. The pathologist examining the tissue that has been removed and determining how many biopsies show cancer and if from one or both sides of the prostate gland does this. Then the urologist must look at the big picture, taking into account the PSA, trends in the PSA levels over time, how many biopsies are positive, how aggressive the cancer appears, and other signs or symptoms.

The next question is, will the cancer kill me? Probably not. This is not a time to panic; it is a time to gather information. Whether or not this cancer will be significant and affect the quality or length of your life depends on a number of factors. Further tests may be necessary before your doctor can decide if the cancer is a threat and how best to respond. Now is the time for you and your doctor to discuss the treatment options and decide what to do next.

GLEASON AND GRADING OF CANCER

As with most cancers, there are various grades of prostate cancer. Some are very aggressive, with the cells looking nothing like original tissues. These are called high-grade, or poorly differentiated. Other cells may resemble normal cells except for a few key points. These are called low-grade, or well differentiated. Most pathologists and urologists use a special grading scale to help standardize prostate cancer evaluation. In this way, doctors across the country can talk about a patient and understand the grade of cancer in question.

The most common grading scale for the comparison of cancers is the Gleason Scale. In this grading system, named after a pathologist, cancer cells are assigned a certain point value based on standard criteria. These criteria describe and rate the cancer cells in two ways: 1) how the cancer cells look, and 2) how they are arranged together. Each component is given a number from 2 to 5, with the sum of the two numbers being the Gleason sum. The urologist may refer to a cancer as a "Gleason 7" or simply "a grade 5." The higher the number, the worse the cancer.

The "Gleason Scale" grades and seeks to predict the tumor's biologic malignancy. It expresses the risk of progression and the probability of death from cancer. Microscopic examination of tumor cells obtained through biopsies reveals five major different but recurring cell patterns. From one to five of these patterns may be found in a specimen. The pathologist identifies the two predominant patterns on a scale of one to five, adds the scales of the two principal patterns together and obtains the final Gleason scale. The grade is based on whether the cancer cells are clearly, individually defined ("differentiated") or irregular, not clearly separate and deferred (not "differentiated"). So, 1 + 1 = 2, the lowest and you might say "best" end of the scale, 5 + 5 = 10, the highest end. Doctors classify a grade of 7 or above as indicative of future trouble, but that, too, depends on other factors. So in practice there are five "scales," the Gleason grade (histological), the stage (A-D), your age, your general health, and the genetic (DNA) makeup of the cancer cells themselves, generally referred to as "ploidy."

Remember that cancer cells are abnormal. They do not behave like the normal cells in the body. Loosely speaking, they present their own DNA patterns. They become independent of the rules of cell birth and death that govern normal cells. It is the growth and independent spread of cancer cells unregulated by normal cell guidelines that make them dangerous.

During the last five years various studies have closely related the Gleason grade with life expectancy; the more undifferentiated the cells, the more dangerous the tumor. Indeed, insurance companies may offer a policy to a prostate cancer survivor whose treatment appears to have been successful, but will hesitate and perhaps refuse insurance if the Gleason tests show poorly differentiated cells, regardless of the clinical (A-D) stage assigned. Discussions of a patient's condition usually include whether his cancer is "differentiated" or "undifferentiated."

Like using cancer volume and the PSA level, the grade of cancer is an important indicator. In fact, all three are related. Larger cancers and higher PSA levels usually mean more aggressive cancer cells. Left untreated, the cancer will continue to grow. As it grows, it will secrete more PSA and the cells will become more aggressive. Like a snowball rolling downhill, the cancer grows faster and faster. This rapid development is why it is important to learn as much as possible by taking the PSA test, a prostate examination, ultrasound findings, and biopsy results to decide what to do and when to do it. Ideally the doctor can use this information to cure you of your cancer during the window of opportunity.

The window of opportunity is the time from the point of discovery of cancer until the time when the cancer begins to spread outside the prostate. During this time, you have more options including choices that are potentially curative, such as radiation and surgery. When the cancer grows outside the prostate, the options will focus on cancer control rather than cure.

I remember after my husband was diagnosed with prostate cancer, Dr. Cohen sat down and discussed treatment options. It is so difficult not to show your emotions when confronted with this type of news, but Dr. Cohen's friendly smile and his reassuring hand on my shoulder somehow broke the nervous tension and put me at ease. But first, he needed to know whether the cancer had spread outside the prostate. He also needed to know the stage of the cancer.

HOW ADVANCED IS THE CANCER

After a CT scan and bone scan is obtained and if this is felt necessary by the urologist the prostate cancer can then be staged, which means predicting whether it is localized or has spread.

Many urologists feel that if the PSA is less than 18, the bone scan and CT scan may not even be necessary because these tests are usually normal when the PSA is below this number and the Gleason grade is less than 7.

There are several tests available to help detect cancer outside the prostate. These tests also provide valuable information about cancer that helps in determining the most appropriate treatments. Whether your doctor recommends a specific test depends on how suspicious he is that the cancer has grown outside the prostate and what information each test can provide.

A bone scan is a nuclear medicine imaging technique in which a tiny amount of radioactive substance is injected into the bloodstream. The nuclear tracer circulates throughout the body and is absorbed by the bones. Certain abnormalities, including cancer, can be determined by this test. The bone scan is the most sensitive imaging technique available today to identify cancer in the bones. The spine is the most common site outside of the pelvis for the spread of prostate cancer. The scan often detects cancer in the bones long before regular x-rays can. The bone scan does not show cancer, but it does show areas of rapid bone growth associated with cancer. Prostate cancer, when it spreads to the skeleton, typically has a classic pattern or random and variable "hot spots" that show up on the scan. This occurs frequently along the spine, ribs, hips and long bones.

The bone scan is used to detect if the prostate cancer has spread to the bones. The spine and other bones are among the most common locations for the spread of prostate cancer. If the bone scan doesn't show anything, it doesn't mean that there is definitely no cancer to the bones, but is a hopeful sign.

STAGING PROSTATE CANCER

Staging means if the cancer is localized or has spread. The urologist uses the PSA; results of CT scan and/or bone scan if obtained to make this determination. There are various stages of prostate cancer; the two common classification systems are the ABCD and the "Whitmore-Jewett" system as well as the TNM staging system.

The ABCD system is as follows.

Stage A - Cancer found incidentally or because of elevated PSA, or during a transurethral resection of the prostate (TURP).

Stage A1 - Is usually a low-grade disease in small volume found incidentally during prostate surgery for BPH.

Stage A2 - When the cancer is high-grade and aggressive or seen in more then 15 percent of prostate tissue removed during a TURP.

Stage A3 - When a cancer is identified because of an elevated PSA alone and a normal rectal exam. Most often these cancers are substantial

Stage B - When cancer is detected because of an irregularity or nodule found during prostate examination.

Stage B1 - When prostate cancer is located on just one side of the prostate.

Stage B2 - When the cancer is on both sides of the gland, but with the evidence of spread outside the gland or to bones or lymph nodes.

Stage C - When the cancer has started to grow locally outside of the gland, but with no spread to bones or lymph nodes (spread may be to the seminal vesicles).

Stage D - When the cancer has spread either to lymph nodes or to the bones.

Stage D1 - When local spread of the cancer to the lymph nodes is confined within the pelvis.

Stage D2 - When cancer has started to spread to the bones.

The TNM staging system provides a more detailed picture of how far the cancer has spread. The report will include a capital T (for tumor) with a number between 1 and 4 and a lower-case letter (a, b or c) next to it. The greater the number and letter, the farther the cancer has spread. For example, a T2c cancer is confined to the prostate but covers more areas of the gland than a T2a cancer. A T3c cancer has spread a little beyond the prostate, while a T4a cancer has spread far beyond the gland. If the lymph nodes contain cancer, the staging report also will include a capital N (for nodes) with a plus sign next to it. "N+." If the cancer has spread beyond the prostate-to the bones, the staging report will include a capital M (for metastasis) with a plus sign next to it "M+." Some doctors use both the ABCD and TNM staging systems, while other doctors use one or the other.

THE TNM CLASSIFICATION TABLE OF PROSTATE CANCER

T	Primary Tumor
T	Primary tumor cannot be assessed
Tx	No evidence of primary tumor
To	Tumor incidental histological finding < 5%
T1a	Tumor incidental histological finding < 5%
T1b	Tumor incidental histological finding > 5%
T1c	Tumor identified by needle biopsy
T2	Tumor confined within the prostate
T2a	Tumor involves one lobe
T2b	Tumor involves both lobes
T3	Tumor extends through prostate capsule
T3a	Extracapsular extension (unilateral/bilateral)
T3b	Tumor invades seminal vesicle(s)
T4	Tumor is fixed or invades adjacent structures
N	Regional lymph nodes
Nx	Regional lymph nodes cannot be assessed
No	No regional lymph node metastasis
N1	Regional lymph node matastasis
M	Distant metastasis
Mx	Distant metastasis cannot be assessed
Mo	No distant metastasis
M1	Distant metastasis
M1a	Non-regional lymph node(s)
M1b	Bone(s)
M1c	Other site(s)

Hormone-naïve
- Never previously having hormonal manipulation

Androgen-dependent
- Having received hormonal manipulation but with less than continuous application, for example, with intermittent androgen blockade or therapy with an agent that does not produce a castrate testosterone level such as with an anti-androgen.

Androgen-independent
- Progressive disease when serum testosterone levels are in the castrate range

Hormone-sensitive
- Patients still may be potentially responsive to other hormone therapy, termed second-line hormone therapy

Hormone-refractory: androgen-independent and hormone-insensitive
- Progressive disease with castrate serum testosterone levels and failure of one or more hormonal manipulations.

TREATMENT OPTIONS
FOR PROSTATE CANCER

Prostate cancer is the most commonly diagnosed cancer among American men and the second leading cause of cancer death among men, making it one of the biggest health concerns in this country. With the widespread use of prostate-specific antigen (PSA)-based screening since the late 1980s, the detection of prostate cancer has risen dramatically. Men now are being diagnosed with prostate cancer at an earlier age and more are being diagnosed when the cancer is confined to the prostate.

With increased patient awareness and widespread PSA screening, the death rate from prostate cancer has decreased significantly. However, metastatic prostate cancer is still found in 20% to 30% of patients with newly diagnosed prostate cancer.

Once diagnosed with prostate cancer, the decision whether, when and how to treat needs to be addressed. The treatment recommended depends upon whether the cancer is localized (confined to the prostate) or metastatic (spread beyond the prostate). Treatment options must also take into consideration other factors including age of the patient, the presenting PSA, aggressiveness of the cancer, the overall health of the patient, and the life expectancy of the patient. What follows is an explanation of the various treatment options for localized and metastatic prostate cancer.

My husband was in the ideal stage for curative treatment, because if you have a normal life expectancy of seven to ten years, radical prostatectomy is probably the best choice.

I remember Dr. Cohen telling me about a number of his patients who incorrectly believed that if they opted for watchful waiting, they could just go home and need not return for follow-up examinations or PSA blood tests. It seems that from 25% to 30% of men with prostate cancer choose "watchful waiting" or observation. This is not without potentially serious risks. In the right patients, observation may well be the best option. For others, though, it can be quite dangerous, because observation means to choose no treatment for the cancer. As Dr. Cohen has often stated to his patients, this obviously depends on a number of factors, age, general health, and family longevity.

The fact is, many men have prostate cancer and are never affected by it during their lifetime. Most don't even know they have prostate cancer. However, it is believed by urologists, like Dr. Cohen, who specialize in prostate cancer, that if prostate cancer is detected because of an abnormality on examinations or because the PSA level is elevated, there is the possibility of significant cancer.

It is always sad when someone chooses a conservative approach only to succumb later to the disease. As much as Dr. Cohen respects his patients' decisions, he always tells them what is the best direction to pursue in dealing with their particular situation. Consequently, Dr. Cohen has been in a class of his own and with an excellent reputation because of his unselfish devotion to his patients. We all know that when someone is diagnosed with an illness requiring surgery-especially upon hearing the word cancer-numbness spills throughout the body. And, the first thought is often, have we chosen the right doctor? It is, therefore, important to receive comfort and assurance that the prospects after surgery look bright. There are many doctors, but it takes a special person to deal with cancer patients requiring surgery.

TREATMENT OPTIONS FOR LOCALIZED PROSTATE CANCER

The most appropriate treatment for localized prostate cancer continues to be debated, as there are still no published randomized trials comparing all treatment options. The physician must provide the best advice based on current data. Treatment options for localized prostate cancer include:

-Watchful waiting

-Radical prostatectomy or surgical removal of the entire prostate gland

-External beam radiation therapy

-Brachytherapy or radioactive seed implantation

-Cryotherapy

WATCHFUL WAITING

Watchful waiting is when a patient with prostate cancer is closely followed with physical examination, including rectal examination and periodic PSA testing.

Most recent studies have shown that untreated men with a life expectancy of 10 to 15 years have a 60% to 80% chance of dying from prostate cancer. This is a new argument against watchful waiting. The conclusions are that watchful waiting is a viable alternative to elderly males, older than 75, with slow-growing cancers. Watchful waiting is not the best option for men in their 50s or 60s with a moderate to fast-growing cancer, since the curability of the cancer may be lost during the waiting period.

SURGERY OPTION

Radical prostatectomy or surgical removal of the entire prostate gland is an operation that has undergone significant refinements over the past 15 years. The operation is now performed in such a fashion as to preserve potency in many patients. The urologist is able to surgically remove the entire prostate gland and reconnect the bladder to the urethra through an incision in the lower abdomen. Usually, a hospital stay of two to three days is required. It has become one of the most common treatments for localized prostate cancer and is considered by many to be the gold standard of treatment to which all other treatments are compared.

The biggest benefit of surgery is that if the cancer is confined to the prostate gland, a cure can be achieved in 96% of patients. The major complications of radical prostatectomy include impotence, incontinence, rectal injury and stricture (scar tissue) formation. The complications of radical prostatectomy continue to fall, with potency being preserved in 40% to 89 % of patients, depending on potency prior to surgery. Significant incontinence is now a rare complication, occurring in only one or two percent of patients. Radical prostatectomy provides the most effective local control of prostate cancer in properly selected patients. Survival after surgery depends upon many factors, but with organ-confined tumors, death from prostate cancer is rare.

EXTERNAL BEAM RADIATION THERAPY

Standard radiation therapy involves 35 to 37 treatments usually administered five days per week for seven to eight weeks. The position of the prostate is determined by bony landmarks, CT scanning and x-rays. A major advance has been the introduction of three- dimensional conformal radiation, where the aim is to conform the radiation to the patient's anatomy, thereby reducing the local side effects. In properly selected patients, conformal radiation can provide excellent cancer control rates. One concern with standard radiation therapy is that post-radiation biopsies two years after treatment showed recurrent or persistent prostate cancer in up to 80% of patients. Recently, hormonal therapy has been used along with external beam radiation therapy in hopes of improving these results.

Side effects of radiation include diarrhea, rectal irritation, frequency and urgency of urination, blood in urine, impotence and, rarely, incontinence.

External radiation therapy is now often used in addition to brachytherapy, to deliver higher-dose radiation to the prostate with fewer side effects and with the goal of increased cure rates. In summary, external radiation therapy is an attractive treatment for patients older than 70 or with life expectancy of less than 10 years.

BRACHYTHERAPY OR RADIATION SEED IMPLANTATION

Historically, brachytherapy or the insertion of radioactive seeds directly into the prostate was first done in the 1950s and again in the 1970s, but was done as an open surgical procedure. The initial results were inferior to external beam therapy and the procedure was abandoned. Since 1985, ultrasound-directed implants allow more precise placement of Iodine-125-seeds without an operation or an incision. Radioactive agents now available for implantation are iodine for slow and moderately aggressive tumors and palladium for the faster, more aggressive cancers.

As technology and knowledge increase, the long-time treatment methods for containing prostate cancers (and for BPH, as we have seen) are being challenged by rapidly developing optional methods. Principal among these are radioactive implants, familiarly called "seeds." Insertion of radioactive materials into the prostate, medically termed brachytherapy, probably started when a Dr. Pasteau inserted radium using a catheter through the urethra. Early trials using radium produced many complications. But the development of new "interstitial implant therapy" techniques and improved radioactive materials stimulated new interest. If the implanted radioactive seeds work well, the patient may avoid some of the problems of recurrence marking external beam radiation (XRT). Also, because of danger of damage to the rectum and bladder from XRT, maximum beam dosages are at their upper limit. Adding implants can almost double the radiation strength without the concurrent damage to nearby healthy tissues.

Dr. Cohen now performs these "seed" implants on many of his patients. Studies now exceed ten years and the results rival those of radical prostatectomy in properly selected patients. Its advantages over XRT and surgery include reduced cost to patients, usually as an outpatient procedure and there usually is quick resumption of normal activities, including sex, in most treatments, reduced radiation risk to medical personnel, and reduced possibility of damage to prostatic adjacent tissues and organs.

Techniques improving interstitial implants include the use of transrectal ultrasound in placing the seeds precisely, and in a pattern designed to make sure all cancerous tissue is bombarded with radioactivity and finding and developing a variety of materials from which to make the seeds. In some instances, external beam treatment may be augmented by permanent seed implantation.

"Seeds" look just like the seeds on rye bread or small grains of rice. With transrectal ultra-sound guidance the seeds are put into place through needles inserted in the prostate. To be effective, they are set from 0.8 to 1 cm (0.32 to 0.4 inches) apart in a three-dimensional grid. Since they don't emit radiation very far from the insertion point, they do not endanger sensitive tissues elsewhere. Fifty to a hundred or more seeds might be inserted in the prostate, depending on the size of the prostate itself and the dose to be delivered.

At about $25 per seed for iodine-125, for example, this is not an inexpensive treatment. Other elements cost more, palladium-103 about twice as much. But bachytherapy costs considerably less than surgery or external beam radiation treatment. A smaller gland will require fewer seeds, but could require a higher strength dose per seed. Dosage is calculated to fit each patient. Seeds are prepared to the radiation strength the physician designates. Seeds are inserted in the patient the day they arrive from the "seed factory." The grid to help arm the needle through which the seeds are placed appears on the ultrasound screen.

The seeds are inserted under ultra-sound guidance using needles placed in the perineal, (the area between the scrotum and the anus). This approach has led to excellent results as compared to the previous approach, which required open surgery placing seeds directly into the prostate.

Seeds might be used as an initial treatment, or in treatment of a previous radiation treatment failure. They are frequently used in conjunction with external beam radiation when bulky tumors are involved so the dosage at the tumor site can be stronger. Either open dissection of lymph nodes or a laparoscopic exam of the nodes may be necessary before seeding, to see if the cancer has spread.

Most implants now being used are permanent. The needle is withdrawn and the seeds remain. When their job is done, they stay in place. Some implants are temporary. These emit higher energies and higher dosages and usually employ an iridium isotope. They remain in place two or three days and are removed in a second procedure.

Dr. Cohen inserts his implants on an outpatient basis under spinal anesthesia. Seeds are guided into predetermined positions with ultra-sound. Some doctors use CT scanning and/or fluoroscopy depending on their respective skills and preferences. All these methods are reported to work well. A high degree of patient acceptance of the procedure was reported and the early favorable PSA response was encouraging. "In this era of cost containment, implant alone offers the potentially least morbid, fastest and least expensive method of treatment for early stage prostate carcinoma," in properly selected patients.

In a limited number of comparison studies made of reports covering different time periods, implantation showed improved reduction of PSA counts over external beam therapy. In a comparison using a small study of surgical patients two years after treatment, implantation appeared almost equal in reducing PSA elevations.

Dr. Cohen has mentioned that the patient's eligibility for the process is evaluated to assure that the cancer is localized to the prostate. The patient also is scheduled for a pre-treatment planning session at which the prostate volume is measured by ultrasound and a grid designed showing where the seeds will be placed. A very large prostate might not be adequately treated especially if a large portion of the prostate is behind the pubic bone, then the implant may not be feasible. Sometimes the prostate size can be reduced with LHRH agonists, such as Lupron, and in some patients the doctors elect to drill holes through the bone in order to place the needle. In others, angled needle placement is possible.

Dr. Cohen always wants to know any medication his patients may be taking. They also undergo the usual hospital pre-op tests, blood counts, EKG, chest X-ray, and urinalysis. A light diet is advised and a laxative is ordered. An anesthesiologist talks with the patient. Usually a spinal or epidural anesthesia is administered. A catheter is inserted into the bladder. The patient is awake or dozing intermittently during the operation. The implant usually takes 30 to 60 minutes and afterward the patient goes to a recovery room. Two hours after the anesthesia wears off, he's ready to go home. He is given an anti-biotic prescription and is advised to take a stool softener. For a time, he is advised to avoid blood-thinning drugs, such as aspirin, Persantine, or Cumadin.

Depending on their type and strength, seeds go on working for an extended time, perhaps three to six months, irradiating cancer and healthy cells alike as the patient goes about his business. The healthy cells can heal, the cancerous ones cannot, and they slough off or are digested by the body. The recovery phase takes nearly a year, which is why it takes so long to appraise the effectiveness of the treatment.

Dr. Cohen has stated that with implants there are mixed complications. The most common side effects are bladder and urethral irritative symptoms, some requiring medication. These symptoms abate within a month for most patients, although some were troubled for four to six months. A few developed urinary retention and required catheterization for several days. In some cases there may be some swelling of the testicles for a short time and some urinary difficulties.

In certain lesions seeds seem to work better and, of course, they are quicker, since they take only one procedure. Seeds also are less expensive, although you don't want your treatment selected on a bargain basis. Using seeds also can save potency possibly 90 to 95 percent of the time. If a patient wants to resume sex immediately, or if he wants to go fishing next week, he might choose seeds over external beam therapy or even surgery. Dr.

Cohen tells of a patient who said, "I want to keep living now. I don't want to worry about when I'm eighty. I'll take my chances on old age." So, treatment can also depend on the patient's outlook.

The best candidates for brachytherapy are patients with small prostate cancers, localized to one side of the prostate, and who have a small to medium-sized prostate gland. External radiation is given four to five weeks before brachytherapy in patients with larger volume or bilateral disease. Side effects of brachytherapy are typically less than those of external radiation but include burning and frequency of urination, rectal irritation, and diarrhea. Incontinence is rare and impotence occurs in less than 25% of patients with brachytherapy alone.

The benefit of brachytherapy is that it is well tolerated as an outpatient procedure. The procedure takes approximately one hour and is performed under regional anesthesia. Normal activity can resume in one to two days. The 10-year data are now available and, with properly selected patients, show very similar disease-free intervals compared to radical prostatectomy, and is superior to external radiation therapy. Brachytherapy is an excellent alternative for older patients because it is better tolerated than surgery or external beam radiation. Younger patients with early low-volume cancers may also be suitable candidates for brachytherapy.

With increased patient awareness and widespread PSA screening, the death rate from prostate cancer has decreased significantly.

CRYOSURGERY

Cryosurgery, or freezing of the prostate gland, has recently been removed from investigational status and is now a covered procedure under most insurance plans. Several centers that perform cryosurgery exist around the country but there are few long-term studies, most being two to four years. Cryosurgery is an alternative treatment option for men with localized prostate cancer and is also used to patients with recurrent or persistent prostate cancer after failed radiation treatment. Important issues, which must be addressed, include patient selection, and the comparison of cost, quality, and cure with existing treatment modalities.

There are several reasons for urology's contained enthusiasm. For one thing, cryosurgery has been used for a quarter of a century in dermatology, gynecology, and other areas, and has proven effective in treating otherwise inoperable liver cancers, for example, among other malignancies. Conversion to liquid-carrying probes instead of nitrogen gas enabled delivery at lower temperatures and more precise and effective control, thus opening the way to treat tissues deep within the body. Earlier cryosurgical procedures used open perineal and abdominal surgical incisions to get to the prostate. This meant more surgery-related after effects in addition to those caused by inadequate freezing.

Other reasons for the optimism are that cryosurgery takes only one to two hours, causes no significant blood loss and fewer side effects than other treatments. It requires only two or three days in the hospital and costs about half as much as radiation or surgical prostate removal. Two or three days after treatment the patient may return to normal physical activities. And for those initially treated by radiation it has the unique capacity in that "armamentarium" to perform as a second or salvage therapy if the cancer recurs.

Cryosurgery may be a significant alternative in dealing with prostate cancer. At least two of the centers in their early use of the five-probe machine tried it on men whose PSAs rose and who showed positive biopsies after radiation. Short-run follow-ups (three to six months) revealed most PSAs down to the 0.2 ng/ml level. Positive biopsies placed the failure rate for the salvage process at 35 %. Tests at other centers confirmed the greater difficulty of salvage cures following radiation. Later trials have produced better results. But if 65 percent of the men who fail radiation can be significantly improved, perhaps even cured of cancer, cryosurgery may be a very positive alternative treatment for patients with prostate cancer.

METASTATIC PROSTATE CANCER

Metastatic prostate cancer is diagnosed when the cancer is found to have spread outside the prostate gland. The most common sites for prostate cancer to spread are to the lymph nodes, bone, liver and lung. Metastatic prostate cancer is predictable if the PSA is greater than 10, and the cancer is of high grade. CT scans diagnoses metastatic prostate cancer and bone scan. Treatment for metastatic prostate cancer is palliative, meaning that its goal is to alleviate symptoms without affecting a cure. Men are treated with a form of hormonal therapy, which treats the entire body putting the cancer in remission in 70 percent to 80 percent of cases. In those men who respond to therapy, the length of time that the tumor remains under control is variable, but can be many years.

Hormonal therapy is used to remove testosterone, the male hormone that allows many prostate cancers to grow. The testicles manufacture almost all of the male hormones, with a small amount also made by the adrenal glands. The testicular production of testosterone can be eliminated by surgically removing the testicles (orchiectomy) or by hormonal injections. (Lupron or Zolodex). Hormonal injections are long-acting drugs, usually given every three to four months, which act on the pituitary gland in the brain. This turns off the testicles' ability to make male hormones.

Side effects of hormone therapy include hot flashes, impotence, mood swings and osteoporosis. Newer approaches to hormone therapy include complete androgen blockade and intermittent hormone therapy, both attempts to prolong the period of remission.

In summary, hormone treatment for metastatic prostate cancer has been used successfully for over 50 years. Initially, 70 percent to 80 percent of patients will respond. Unfortunately, the response is rarely permanent and usually within two to five years after starting hormone treatment the cancer will no longer respond and will start to grow again.

This, of course, highlights the importance of early diagnosis and treatment of prostate cancer before it spreads outside the gland.

Men who have been diagnosed with prostate cancer have several categories of treatment from which to choose when discussing this with their physician. Each choice has definite pros and cons and, therefore, each patient should carefully think through each option.

It should be noted that it is difficult to decide what treatment is best for you based on the clinical stage of cancer alone, since many factors that cannot be addressed here must enter into your decision regarding treatment.

First, however, each patient should compare the risks with the long-term benefits. The more risks you take today, the more potential for the best long-term results. The reason for this is that, in general, the more aggressive the treatment, the better the chances for cure. But the aggressive treatments are more risky for the patient.

WHAT IS THE RIGHT TREATMENT?

When prostate cancer is diagnosed, deciding on the type of treatment for each patient is the bottom line question. As Dr. Cohen has mentioned many times, if we could know what each patient's future holds and what is really going on in his prostate, then the answers would be easy. However, no one knows what tomorrow holds for any of us.

It is interesting to note that with prostate cancer, everyone expects the doctors to have all the answers and know the "right" course of treatment for each individual. Here it depends on what you have chosen to do for your prostate cancer. If you have chosen to do nothing and there is evidence that the cancer has spread, then you still may be able to opt for the choices previously discussed. If you have chosen surgery as a treatment, you have the option of changing your mind right up until the day of surgery. However, if you are having second thoughts, then you should talk with your doctor right away. But, if you have started radiation, you should finish all the treatments.

Many patients have asked, "Dr. Cohen, how long can I take to choose a treatment?" There really is not a time limit. You should take the time to gather the information you need to make an intelligent decision. Avoid, if possible, snap decisions. Most of Dr. Cohen's patients decide within a few weeks what treatment they wish to pursue. Remember that if you choose surgery, there will be a delay of three to four weeks while you donate your blood so that it will be available if needed during your surgery. However, some patients choose to postpone treatment due to prior commitments for personal reasons. If it is a delay of a few months, then it probably will not make any difference how far the cancer will progress during that time. Bear in mind, however, there is no way to know for certain, and there are no guarantees.

If you are going to postpone treatment for several months or more, then you may want to consider getting hormone shots once a month to keep the cancer in check. Although controversial, some would encourage pre-treatment with three months of hormones to shrink the prostate gland and make the surgery easier or the radiation more effective. Always remember that there are no guarantees the cancer will not spread during a significant delay of treatment. We do know that the higher the PSA the more aggressive the cancer. We also know that the more volume of cancer seen, the more likely the cancer is going to, or has already started to, grow through the capsule or spread to other sites.

If you have questions or concerns about your disease or your treatment options, you should consider getting a second medical opinion before you make a final decision. With prostate cancer, you have time to think about treatments and to seek additional opinions. Many insurance companies require a second opinion, although this is often waived for cancer treatment and surgery.

Be aware that some doctors may feel insulted or hurt if, after spending an hour or more going over all the details and options, you say you want a second opinion. It is most important to tell your doctor that you appreciate the time and effort given and that you respect and trust his opinion. But make it clear that before you finalize your decision, you would like to speak with another urologist and/or radiation therapist. Dr. Cohen always encourages speaking to as many other specialists as you need in order to feel comfortable prior to making a decision. Dr. Cohen also encourages his patients to talk with their primary care physician as well.

URINARY INCONTINENCE

Urinary incontinence is the involuntary loss of urine. In simpler terms, it is leaking urine when you do not know that you are or when you are not trying to. This condition can be a temporary or permanent side effect of treatments for prostate cancer. The key to bladder control is a combination of the circular muscle fibers at the bladder neck and the sphincter muscles located beneath the bladder surrounding the urethra. This muscle combination works to close off the urethra and prevent leakage of urine from the bladder. When the prostate is removed from the base of the bladder, damage can occur to the urinary sphincter that gives men a mechanism for holding in urine naturally. This damage can result in incontinence. There are various surgical techniques for operating on this anatomy during a prostatectomy, but the danger of tissue and muscle damage is ever present.

The Kegel exercise is simply an exercise to strengthen the pelvic muscles. As a group of muscles, they can be exercised and trained to be stronger. That is the reason Dr. Cohen encourages the Kegel exercise for men who will undergo radical prostatectomy. After surgery, while the catheter is in place, it is important to continue working the pelvic muscles. Dr. Cohen has had patients tell him that when they stopped the exercises, they noticed a dramatic increase in incontinence.

As Dr. Cohen has mentioned to his patients they probably already are doing this exercise unknowingly. As an example, when you are urinating and suddenly stop midstream - that is the Kegel exercise. Also if you are standing in a public place and suddenly feel the urge to pass gas, and you "snug up" the muscles to hold it in, that too is the Kegel exercise. Dr. Cohen described it as a tightening of the pelvic muscles.

In time, many men can relearn how to use the muscles weakened during surgery. Dr. Cohen strongly encourages his patients to begin practicing their sphincter tightening exercises even before surgery. These are simple exercises to strengthen the pelvic muscles. This is the reason we encourage Kegel exercise for men who will undergo radical prostatectomy.

Many probably already do this exercise unknowingly. When you are urinating and suddenly stop midstream that is the Kegel exercise. This would best be described as a tightening of the pelvic muscles. No one around you will know you are doing these exercises if you are doing them correctly.

You need to do them regularly, not just when you think of it. Dr. Cohen suggested twenty Kegels four to five times a day, holding each for two to three seconds. When the catheter is removed, you should be doing the exercises at least one hundred times a day. It is important that you don't just tighten up and then let go. Rather, tighten up and hold it, then let go and repeat. Don't just do it as an exercise. Before surgery and after the catheter comes out, practice stopping midstream when you urinate. Hold it and then restart forcefully. This should help build up and restore the muscle tone. You should continue to do these exercises as long as you have a problem with urinary leakage. This could be a few days to a few months. In rare cases, men may have to do them forever.

There is no way to predict who will leak and who will not, or for how long. Some men claim they never leaked after the catheter came out, while most describe a few weeks to a few months or more of leakage. A few patients have complained of continued leakage for more than a year. If the leakage goes on for a rather long time, this does not mean that it will never stop. In fact, some of Dr. Cohen's patients have reported continued leakage to some degree for several months before everything "dried up." He mentioned that one patient continued with some incontinence for approximately eighteen months. It is important to remember not to become discouraged after a few weeks.

Also remember that leaking does not mean that something was done wrong during surgery. It is simply a reflection of how your body healed. Dr. Cohen recalled that some patients who had successful surgery, still ended up with some incontinence. Then there have been others who had problems in surgery that left the doctor expecting leakage, and they were as dry as a man can be after the catheter came out. Dr. Cohen has had patients who had absolutely no incontinence after the Foley catheter was removed. In fact, one patient wasn't worried until he played golf with several other men who had also had prostate cancer surgery. In sharing their experiences and problems, he came to believe that he was supposed to leak. He felt sure something must be wrong. Dr. Cohen had to reassure him during a post-operative check-up that all was well and that he was one of the fortunate ones.

A question often asked after radical prostatectomy surgery is," Are there any medications that can help?" Certain medications and decongestants such as Entex LA and Ornade help to tighten the urethral muscles and may reduce urine leakage. However, since these medications can increase your blood pressure, it is a good idea to have your blood pressure checked possibly twice a week. There also is a device called the Cunningham penile clamp, which snaps onto the penis and prevents urine leakage. But if used at all, it should be used only for short periods of time. If left on the penis too long, damage to the skin and underlying tissues can occur. Dr. Cohen has discouraged men from using a clamp in the first few months after surgery. He has seen a few patients who have become totally dependent on the clamp. These men stop trying to regain control, and since they no longer do the Kegel exercises, they remain incontinent. The penile clamp applies direct physical pressure to the urethra, forcing it to shut so there is no leakage of urine. It is important to take this clamp off about every thirty minutes to let your bladder empty and then reapply as needed. This will also allow the blood flow to keep tissues healthy. These patients are advised to use the clamp only for special occasions, such as going out to dinner, the movie or to church. Problems could arise if the clamp is used too early after surgery, or too often, since you will not be motivated to work on controlling leakage with Kegal exercises. This excessive reliance can result in permanent problems in controlling your urine. Patients are told to wait at least six to eight weeks after surgery before using medications or a Cunningham clamp.

There also are adult male undergarments. These are simply large absorbent underpants, often with a hole cut in which the man places his penis. These work by absorbing any urine that leaks. These garments are usually used in the early phases of recovery after surgery.

There are operations to correct incontinence. If the leakage is severe and prolonged, the urologist can operate to place a device called an artificial sphincter. This is a device made from silicone-based materials. It is surgically placed around the urethra, just at the bladder neck. When activated by a pump in the scrotum, this device tightens around the urethra and prevents urine from leaking. This procedure usually takes several hours under anes-thesia. There is usually at least an overnight stay in the hospital. However, it is important to have a complete evaluation before surgery to be sure there is normal bladder function and no scarring or other irregularities that may compromise the results. A cystoscopy is usually done to evaluate the bladder neck visually.

Problems can occur with an artificial sphincter because this is an operation with implantation of a mechanical device and one must be aware that there are risks of failure or problems. Some of these problems include bleeding, infection around the device, urinary retention, continued incontinence, and malfunction or breakage of the artificial sphincter. Although rare, these problems can occur. Only a small percentage of men need additional surgery to adjust the device or repair any malfunction. It is impor-tant to be aware of how this device works so you will have real-istic expectations. Also, since it is a mechanical device, a low percentage of malfunctions are expected. This could require addi-tional surgery.

Patients have asked whether there are any other procedures to overcome incontinence. The answer is yes. In fact, many men are having injections of collagen into the bladder neck to reduce leakage. The collagen is injected through a flexible needle into the tissues at the bladder neck. When successful, this causes the tissues to enlarge and squeeze together to prevent leakage. Collagen is the protein extract of connective tissue from cattle. It is injected elsewhere in the body by plastic surgeons as a filler to add shape or fullness. Five to seven sessions of collagen injections may be required to achieve control of urine. There is no way to know in advance how many times a person will need treatment. Most injections are performed under general anesthesia, but can be done under local anesthesia.

If the collagen works, it should be effective for at least a few years. Some men will notice that it gradually becomes less effective over several years. Each individual may have different results. Some may have great urinary control for several months and then notice increased leaking. Others may go many years without problems. Remember, however, collagen injections do not work for everyone. In fact, as a treatment for urine leakage after a radical prostatectomy, perhaps only a third of patients may notice some improvement. But collagen injections are easy to do as an outpatient procedure and can be repeated. You also need to have tests before collagen injection treatments because a possible side effect is an allergic reaction. Therefore, a skin test is required at least three to four weeks before the collagen treatment. Basically, the test involves an injection of a tiny amount of collagen under the surface of the skin of your arm. If you are allergic to collagen, you will get a reaction in your arm-redness and firmness, with possible fevers or aches. The chances of an allergic reaction to collagen injections are very rare, but because they can be serious, special precautions must be taken.

IMPOTENCE

Impotence and problems with erections are potential side effects that can result from various treatments for prostate cancer. With few exceptions, if you develop prostate cancer, you will have to consider the impact of the treatments on your ability to have an erection. For those men who already have lost the ability, there is a lot of interest in regaining their potency.

Impotence is the inability to achieve and sustain an adequate erection for sexual intercourse. Erectile dysfunction is the ability to achieve an erection, but it may not be as adequate as you might like. Your penis might be erect, but the erection may not last long enough. In essence, erectile dysfunction is a broader term than impotence.

When one has prostate cancer, erections can be affected since all aspects of prostate cancer and treatments can somehow have an impact on erections. Surgery and radiation can damage the nerves and blood vessels that allow men to achieve and maintain an erection. However, the good news is that with all the new and exciting non-surgical methods of restoring erections, almost everyone can be happy with the final outcome.

If a man chooses to do nothing for his prostate cancer, he could still become impotent. It may be that as the cancer grows and spreads, it can damage the nerves that are just outside the gland. Or perhaps it is a result of fears, concerns, anxiety, and stress that can go along with prostate cancer. Radiation can also make you impotent. Twenty-five to 50 percent of men who undergo radiation therapy will become impotent. Unlike after surgery, where impotence is immediate, impotence after radiation may occur slowly, over months or years. Even if you have great erections before, during, and after radiation treatments, many men describe a slow loss of erections over about one year's time. It is believed to be a result of radiation injury to the small blood vessels and nerves.

Erectile problems can develop after interstitial seed therapy. Up to eighty percent of men who have good erections before treatment will maintain adequate erections afterward. Like external beam therapy, seed therapy can take a while to cause loss of erections. Sometimes radical surgery can actually make a man impotent. Many times the tiny nerves that transmit messages to get an erection can be cut or damaged when removing the prostate. If the message can't get to the penis to allow blood in, there will be no erections. In addition, there may be injury to the blood supply required for erections.

It is still possible to be impotent if you have the nerve-sparing radical prostatectomy. Remember, even if the nerves are saved, it still can take many months for men to regain the ability to have an adequate erection. If only one side of the nerves was saved, then the odds of regaining potency are not great, but it can still happen. This delay may be a result of injury to the nerves during their preservation. Nerves are very slow to heal. Younger, healthier men with good erections are far more likely to have the return of their erections after surgery or radiation than older men who already had erection problems.

If one suffers from erectile disfunction after prostate surgery, there are multiple non-invasive as well as minimally invasive treatments. Perhaps the most popular first option is medication, and here Viagra leads the way. Taken one hour before relations it can increase blood flow to the penis during stimulation, and has success rates of forty percent in men after prostate cancer treatment. The only definite contra-indication to using Viagra is if one has heart disease and is taking nitroglycerine.

If medical treatment fails, the next least invasive treatment would be a vacuum system-an external device to increase blood to the penis. Other options include penile injections or intra-utheral suppository to dilate penile blood vessels and increase blood supply to the penis. If these minimally invasive treatments fail, a penile prosthesis can be surgically implanted. There are various types both semi-rigid and inflatable, and both carry high patient and partner satisfaction profiles. Talk to your doctor if you are having erectile dysfunction so he can work with you in picking a treatment that will get you back to having the sexual lifestyle that you and your partner deserve.

WIFE'S ROLE

Many times after your doctor tells you that you have prostate cancer, it is not uncommon to forget to involve your wife in the long process of cancer evaluation, treatment, recovery, and life after treatment. Whatever path you choose, and no matter what happens, she will have to watch it from the sidelines.

I remember the look I gave Jim after he made the decision to have surgery. I do not know who was more nervous or upset, Jim or me, but he did make the decision, and, since we both had such confidence in Dr. Cohen, it eased our fears. Always remember, a wife has to live with the results of her husband's decision. I sometimes felt it would be easier to be the patient, because then you are aware of what is happening every step of the way.

When you first go to your urologist, then all the appointments, tests, waiting for results, long discussions about treatment options and controversies, treatment, recovery period, and beginning your life again-hopefully cured-there is your ever-loving wife. I remember quietly sitting and waiting, always trying to stay calm, to be a support to my husband-while an almost overwhelming fear of the unknown silently tormented me.

Women usually do well in times of crisis and serve as the stable pillar for the family during their illness. Your wife also may function as your around-the-clock nurse when problems occur at home. Men should think about this and take the time to include their wives in the decision-making. Just remember some of these questions. Ask her what she thinks. What sounds good? What scares her? Bring her with you to talk to your doctors. Take her to the hospital when you go for pre-operative testing. Most important, give her an opportunity to ask questions. Let her know that her input is important and listen to what she has to say. In many of these situations, some women tend to have more common sense and a better ability to step back and look at the total picture. Remember, prostate cancer is a very personal disease. From the moment your cancer is identified until it is either cured or controlled, it is most essential that men include their wives. And share your feelings with her. Openly discuss your fears and concerns with her about how this might affect your sexual relationship. However, in this day and age, Dr. Cohen will give you many alternatives. You may find that this issue is less important to her than making you well and extending your life. Dr. Cohen, always compassionate, encouraged his patients to bring their wives or companions with them to their appointments.

On the other side, some wives do not feel it is their place to participate in the discussions or decision-making regarding their husband's care. I remember vividly Dr. Cohen, in his soft-spoken voice, telling me that all he can do is try to include the patient's wife. However, if she will not participate in the discussion, she should be encouraged at least to listen so she can better understand what is happening to her husband.

Also, whenever someone is diagnosed with prostate cancer, the decision to tell friends or neighbors about it depends on his relationship with them. I well remember Dr. Cohen's words of caution, in reality, about human nature and cancer. For reasons that no one really understands, he said, whenever the word gets out that you have been diagnosed with prostate cancer, anyone who has had prostate cancer or knows of someone with cancer will seek you out and tell you his horror story. Even if it's not prostate cancer, they feel it is their responsibility to tell you how miserable someone was after radiation for breast cancer, or how many problems someone had with their prostate cancer. Dr. Cohen has strong feelings about these "friendly" bits of advice. This can have some very damaging effects on your morale. As he mentioned, treatments for any disease in the past have nothing to do with treatments today. Even radical prostatectomy, which is surgery to remove the cancerous prostate gland and surrounding tissues, has very much improved. The operation men have today has significantly better results and is much better tolerated than the same operation several years ago.

My husband Jim, who had a radical prostatectomy, was discharged after three days. Dr. Cohen remarked that he did so well that he was inclined to discharge him in two days, but was concerned over what his colleagues would say! Early on, a patient normally was in intensive care for approximately one to two days followed by another five to seven days of hospitalization. Remember, everyone responds differently to treatments. The best thing that you can do when talking to others is to take everything they say with a grain of salt, smile, thank them for their concern, and file the information away. If you are worried, discuss it with your urologist.

Always remember, when a man is faced with prostate surgery-or any surgery for that matter, his wife, who is his best friend and companion will always be there to give the support, love, and understanding you need.

HMOs

Health Maintenance Organizations (HMOs) have grown increasingly popular over the last few years as millions of seniors, lured by low costs and promises of a more comprehensive coverage, have switched from traditional fee-for-services Medicare. Medicare HMOs are less expensive than the traditional fee-for-service Medicare since you do not need to buy supplemental Medigap insurance. While you must continue to pay your Medicare Part B premium-currently $43.80 per month-you will no longer have to pay Medicare deductibles or co-insurance and you won't have to deal with Medicare paperwork.

Some Medicare HMOs don't require any additional monthly premiums, but usually charge a small co-payment for each doctor's visit. In addition to lower costs, you usually have access to extra benefits such as eyeglasses, hearing aids, some prescriptions drug coverage, and dental care. While Medicare HMOs are definitely cheaper, there are tradeoffs. Since HMOs hold down their costs by controlling access to care, they are not always appropriate for older people with chronic health problems who have certain doctors they may want to continue seeing. HMO enrollees must use specific doctors and facilities affiliated with a managed care network and usually must obtain a referral from their primary care physician to see a specialist or to be admitted to a hospital (except in an emergency). Some HMOs offer a point-of-service option whereby you can go out of the network for an additional fee, but those fees can add up if you go outside the system. If you travel extensively or if you are a "snowbird," a Medicare HMO is probably not for you. If you stay outside an HMO's service area for more than three months, you risk losing your coverage.

One of the major attractions of HMOs is their prescription drug coverage. Medicare does not pay for medications and only some of the more expensive Medigap policies do. But, before you sign up for a Medicare HMO in hopes of cutting your drug costs, you need to ask some tough questions about the specific medications that are available.

The abrupt closing of an HMO in New Jersey may be a harbinger of what is to come for millions of HMO users. Here is a case that really happened and why it could happen to you.

Right before a certain individual was diagnosed with prostate cancer, he learned that in just seven weeks, he would be losing his health insurance. It wasn't because this seventy-three-year-old person had failed to pay his premiums, forgotten to fill out the proper paperwork, or missed some vital deadline; it was because the New Jersey Department of Banking and Insurance announced that on March 31 it would be shutting down this individual's HMO. This news left approximately 200,000 consumers scrambling to find new health coverage and to wrap up key medical decisions before the HMO closed its doors. But it also highlighted the shocking financial instability of many of the nations health plans, and warned that there may be more large-scale managed cared failures in the months to come.

The contagion is spreading. One of HMO's New Jersey sister plans, the famed HMO New York, has been financially damaged by the debacle; another HMO ceased operations on April 30. And in California regulators announced in mid-March that they had seized control of the local operations of Med Partners Provider Networks, a physician management group that through contracts with HMOs and other insurance carriers, serves approximately 1.3 million state residents. This year, large established companies that should not be vulnerable to failure are taking hits at an unprecedented rate.

But the financial pressures facing all HMOs stemming from rising pharmaceutical costs, public insistence on additional services, and the plan's inability to raise rates have become so powerful that even the big names can be at risk. This is not just any business failing, for when an HMO fails, people's lives are at stake.

Another case in point: recently a urologist learned that his medical supply company would no longer maintain his stock of chemotherapy drugs because an HMO in New Jersey was delinquent on the bill. And so this doctor, worried about interrupting his patients' treatment, wrote prescriptions for some of his patients who then had to go to the pharmacy, shell out a $9 co-payment for their chemotherapy drugs, and bring them back to his office. That's a horrible complication for someone fighting cancer. As a result, this doctor spent countless hours trying to track down a new supplier and, in some cases, even purchased the drugs himself.

Sometimes, making the transition is likely to prove trying, to say the least. A newly diagnosed prostate cancer patient said he considered letting a doctor closely monitor his tumor's growth, but because he wasn't sure about what kind of care his new health plan would allow, he decided to begin radiation treatments immediately. This individual stated he was worried that the plan he ended up with wouldn't let him see a specialist as often as he felt he should. This seemed to be the safest decision to make, he thought. But was it the best decision? As more and more HMOs find themselves nearing the point of collapse, an increasing number of Americans may soon have their own reasons to wonder.

GRATEFUL SURVIVORS

Going for surgery is never easy, especially if you have been diagnosed with prostate cancer. Just hearing the word "cancer" puts a chill up your spine. Now, what do you do faced with a serious problem and, more importantly, have you chosen the right doctor to help you?

It takes a certain type of personality and skill as a surgeon to deal with cancer patients. There is so much emotion and fear in them because many cancer patients are misinformed, having little or no knowledge of their problem. Support groups are wonderful for anyone with prostate problems or cancer in general; it helps to hear from survivors with problems like their own.

I remember well when one of Dr. Cohen's colleagues was the guest speaker at a support group and spoke on prostate surgery. Dr. Cohen had just joined the urological group at the hospital and was quickly being recognized as a very skilled cancer surgeon specializing in prostate cancer. Dr. Cohen's colleague stated how he had performed radical prostatectomy operations for several years, but when this young, talented, and skilled surgeon had come on board, with such a good reputation from many of his patients, it was decided that Dr. Cohen would handle all radical prostatectomy operations. One of the survivor's stories you are about to hear deals with someone who never had any problems, yet was diagnosed with prostate cancer. Shortly thereafter, he was operated on for radical prostatectomy and today, at Dr. Cohen's urging, started and continues to run a large support group at the hospital here in Palm Beach Country at Wellington Regional Medical Center.

Again, when reading these survivors' stories, keep in mind prostate cancer is known as the "silent disease."

In September of 1991, Alexis Adams saw the advertisement for Wellington Regional Medical Center's free annual prostate screen. She called and made an appointment for her husband, Ash. Ash reluctantly came at his scheduled time. He felt fine and did not really want to have this kind of test. More than two hundred men participated in this screening, consisting of both the PSA laboratory test and a digital rectal examination. Dr. Ross Cohen, urologist, was the physician who examined him. The physical revealed a nodule on the prostate gland His PSA was drawn and sent to the laboratory. His PSA came back elevated. Both Mr. and Mrs. Adams became very concerned. Further diagnostic work-up was immediately ordered.

First, Ash had to have a transrectal ultra-sound and biopsy. The ultra-sound is a painless procedure used to identify and esti-mate the size of both cancerous and non-cancerous conditions. It can also be used in conjunction with a biopsy, as in his case. The biopsy usually causes little or no discomfort. The tests revealed that Ash did indeed have cancer of the prostate. Both he and his wife were devastated and their lives were about to change.

Ash spent the next few weeks having a variety of other tests. He also had a bone scan and a CT scan to see if the cancer had spread outside the prostate. Both tests came back negative. After discussing all the options, Dr. Cohen performed a radical prostate-ctomy on Ash. A tumor approximately the size of a grapefruit was removed.

Ash had absolutely no prior symptoms. As Dr. Cohen mentioned, this is not uncommon, since prostate cancer is a "silent disease," meaning it often causes no noticeable problems until the disease has spread. After successful surgery, Ash has returned to a healthy and productive life. Without question, he has received a second chance and it is difficult to put into words how thankful he is to his loving wife. He is extremely grateful for the support he received from his whole family, but it is because of the skill of Dr. Cohen that he has been given the "gift of life" a second chance.

This individual was in his late 50s when his problems developed. In July of 1997 her husband was very fortunate to have chosen Dr. Cohen as his physician. He was told he had cancer and, needless to say, they both were beside themselves. They remembered how compassionate and upbeat Dr. Cohen was with them, putting them both at ease and allowing them to breathe more easily.

When Dr. Cohen used the cystoscope to check the prostate for invasion, he asked if this person had been doing the exercises he told him to do. He answered, "yes." Then Dr. Cohen wanted to know if they were hard to do. When there was no response, the doctor jokingly said " just because you have a camera up your penis is no reason to go *brain-dead* on me!" This brought smiles to their faces. At this point there was so little to smile about, just joy that the cancer was caught in the early stages. Later this individual asked his primary doctor why he had not checked his PSA or not done the digital examination on him. No comment. After surgery Dr. Cohen gave this individual a ninety-five percent cure. As a result, this person has a new primary care physician, but Dr. Cohen will always have his thanks and praise forever.

Another individual, also in his fifties, attended the prostate cancer support group at Wellington Hospital for prostate cancer and was very interested. This gentleman went for a routine physical with his primary physician. During the examination the doctor detected something on the right side of his prostate and suggested that he see a urologist pending the outcome of his PSA test. He referred this person to a urologist that was on his HMO for an examination. His PSA test came back 7.0 and naturally he became concerned. Up to this point he had no symptoms associated with prostate disease. The urologist concurred with the opinion of his primary doctor and recommended the ultrasound and biopsy that he agreed to have done as soon as possible.

When he arrived at the urologist's office for this exam, this person stated he did not think he had ever been more frightened or pessimistic in his life. He had not slept the night before, and, fortunately, a good friend accompanied him to the examination. His apprehension and fears were not in vain, and regardless of all those who told him it was not going to be a painful experience, he was in near shock. He believes to this day that physicians should administer this test with a mild sedation or anesthetic. This individual went into mild shock and broke out in cold sweats and had to terminate the test after getting only five samples. This doctor was indifferent to his discomfort and fear, but worried that he would upset the patients waiting in the outer office.

"I remained there for approximately twenty minutes until my color returned and was then released." A week later he returned to learn the results. The doctor told him he had a malignant tumor on his prostate. While telling this to him, this doctor continued looking out the window and almost recited the options. He did not seem concerned that he was giving a death sentence. The patient was escorted out and told to return to set up a surgery date. This patient was devastated-a week before Christmas and he had received news that he had cancer.

The thoughts of an operation and a horrible death loomed over him for almost a week. He had never been hospitalized, never operated on, and was sure if he opted for surgery, he would not come out of it. After the holidays, the urologist set him up for an MRI and bone scans to see if the cancer had spread. The results were negative; it was confined to the prostate. Thank God, he thought, for small favors.

Then he saw the advertisement for the meeting of the support group at Wellington Regional with Dr. Cohen the guest speaker. He had heard from a nurse at J. F. Kennedy Hospital that Dr. Cohen had operated on her husband for prostate cancer and had incurred some complications. This nurse further said that Dr. Cohen was at her husband's bedside around the clock until he was sure he was well on the road to recovery. Now he wanted to hear for himself what this doctor had to say regarding treatment for this disease. This is his story:

"The meeting was packed and I saw a young doctor, very confident, outgoing, and not dodging any of the direct questions from the group. His charisma changed my attitude and I resolved to make an appointment with him at the earliest possible time. The meeting took place in his office and he never seemed to be rushed or concerned with anything but my questions, and my concern for the post-surgical problems such as incontinence and impotency. My decision was made, we shook hands, and I felt a weight lifted from my shoulders. He told me that I was a good candidate and should have no problems recovering fully in a short time.

"The date was set, but then arrangements were made for me to donate some of my own my blood, three pints in three weeks. I felt this was really a negative-to have to wait after making a difficult decision, since it would have been a lot easier to go in the next day and get it over with, but the blood is a concern. During this time you pray a lot. Three days prior to the surgery, I reported to pre-op for tests and instructions to follow prior to arriving at the hospital. All of the staff at Wellington Regional were very considerate and told me that I was in very good hands with Dr. Cohen. They further told me that he was a no-nonsense surgeon and very punctual.

"Surgery was scheduled for 8:00 a.m., and before I could get myself upset, I was on the gurney headed for the operating room. I was hospitalized for three days and must honestly say I do not remember any pain. However, I knew I was catheterized and would remain catheterized for about three weeks. This I dreaded more than anything because it looked like a very restricting and uncomfortable thing to be carrying around. One thing about Dr. Cohen, even if there were something wrong, you would never know it from his demeanor. He is always upbeat and optimistic and he will tell you up-front about everything, good, bad or indifferent. The first week of my recovery, I was a real pain in the butt to Dr. Cohen since I had forgotten everything he had said regarding the recovery. However, he always returned my calls. After he removed the catheter, I became a bigger pain and wanted to know when I would stop needing the pads and when would the incontinence stop. Honestly, I learned to cope, do my exercises, and I am about ninety-five percent back to where I should be.

"What a person and what can I say about this physician? I was so pessimistic about today's doctors, the entire health care system, and especially the insurance companies dictating what treatment one gets. Well, Dr. Cohen is a bright light at the end of a very dark tunnel, and I am so grateful that I had the opportunity to meet this talented physician that night when he spoke to the support group and later saved my life."

This man came all the way from Colts Neck, New Jersey, to have his prostate surgery done by Dr. Cohen after he was highly recommended to him as a talented surgeon: "Thank you for all that you have done for me in connection with my recent prostate surgery. Your thoroughness, kindness, gentle manner and spirit of cooperation were greatly appreciated by my family and me. After very successful surgery, I was only in the hospital for four days. My recuperation time also was great. I still have some problems with incontinence, which I am sure will pass soon. You will always be, not only a friend, but a skilled doctor who I will never forget that gave me a second chance to visit Florida as a person again."

This person came from Detroit, Michigan: "From the time my doctor sent me to you until last week when you took the last blood test, you have shown true compassion and professionalism in your field. As we went along, you answered all our questions and later answered all our phone calls in short order. You never ever kept us in the dark. I am sure that there are other doctors out there that could have performed the same prostate operation, but I don't think any one of them would have had the bedside manner you have shown my wife and me. You are truly a dedicated doctor and a true gentleman! For saving my life, you will always have my deepest thanks."

This man came from Boston, Massachusetts: "I feel it is my duty to write this letter praising Dr. Ross Cohen who convinced me during my illness that it was not necessary to go to John Hopkins for my prostate operation. He was so right! I am so glad that we were able to get together. I am also sure my operation was a success due to the skilled hands of Dr. Cohen. It could not have been different if I had the operation at John Hopkins, but he was more than capable. Many thanks for the likes of Dr. Ross Cohen. My thoughts are certainly more positive of the medical profession in South Florida with men like him. He is a boon to the Hippocratic oath."

"Dear Dr. Cohen: You made my life again! I can pee like an old racehorse again. It feels so good. In fact, I never knew that to pee was a miracle. I love you for being so kind and understanding with all my heart and making my life so great again."

"Dear Dr. Cohen and Team: Good morning everybody! I hope you all had a good night's rest before starting this operation. I want you to know that it is very gratifying for me to lie here sleeping with the knowledge that when I wake up my prostate and the cancer in it will be gone. This is all due to your special skills and the accomplished hands of Dr. Cohen. Whatever each of you get paid, you are certainly worth it. Anyway, I guess it's time for you to go to work. Please try to make sure that my penis is left in good working order. Believe it or not, I still use it! Thanks again for all you have done to make me well again."

"Dear Dr. Cohen: I am writing to say 'thank you' for the skill in which you performed my vasectomy and the professionalism displayed by your staff from the moment I called for an appointment. Your staff answered all my questions in a very courteous and patient manner over the telephone before my visit. When I walked through the door for my appointment, I was greeted warmly and with respect as opposed to the usual treatment of 'just another patient.' As for the procedure, you did a great job. I could not believe it was all over in 15 minutes and with very minimal discomfort. I drove home the same day, rested for about four hours and was able to go to work the next morning. I am so glad I chose you to perform the surgery and will highly recommend your practice to all my associates and friends." (He was an executive vice-president of a large manufacturing company.)

My husband, Jim, and I each year took our annual physical examinations at Local Union #3 IBEW in Flushing, New York. At this time Jim received a PSA test. He had no knowledge nor had ever heard of this test, because the medical department always performs many blood tests, and this was the first time the PSA was included (1993). At this time, he did not know what a prostate gland was or its purpose.

The medical department tried in vain to contact us after receiving the blood test results. We had been doing some extensive traveling, but they finally caught up with us by leaving a message at my brother's home. Jim immediately called the union and got in touch with the medical department. They informed him that they had received the results of the blood tests and he was told that his PSA registered 9.5. Jim found out that anything over 4.1 was suspect of being cancerous and that he should consult with a urologist as soon as we returned home.

We had just relocated to Florida and were not familiar with doctors in the urological field. Since I was doing volunteer work at the local hospital, I decided to question people there about names of reputable surgeons in the urological sector. I repeatedly heard one name. "Helen, there is only one doctor you want to take your husband to and his name is Dr. Ross Cohen. He is very demanding, very punctual, but also an excellent surgeon." "We are sure that if surgery is necessary, you will be happy knowing your husband is in the excellent hands of Dr. Cohen." So Jim made an appointment with the urological group that Dr. Cohen was associated with. He was given a rectal examination and they took another blood test that resulted in a PSA reading of 10. Jim was then told to come back for a more extensive rectal examination, and during this exam they were able to snip a piece of tissue from the prostate to send for a biopsy. At this point, Jim heard the doctor and technician discussing the test. He found out that the doctor had seen a small cyst on the left side of his prostate and what appeared to be a little calcium on the right side. The technician agreed and the doctor snipped a sample from the left side. This test was not painful, but a bit uncomfortable.

A few days later, Jim was called to come in for the biopsy result; it was malignant. What a blow to both of us! Jim was a guy who was the picture of health, always felt great, rarely ever caught a cold or took a pill. Now, he finds out he has the big "C," which is an extremely horrible word. Fortunately, I was with him at this meeting and all subsequent meetings, tests, et cetera. He knew I was his pillar and his confidante and still am.

After the shock wore off, we began to discuss treatments and alternative. For the first time we met Dr. Ross Cohen. On our first encounter with him, we were suspicious and wary. Here is this doctor sitting across from us with a spike hair cut and a short beard, looking no older than our son. First impressions!

However, by the end of our meeting we knew the doctor was friendly, compassionate, understanding, and an extremely competent professional. Dr. Cohen said that Jim had four options. First, receive outside radiation; second, seed implants which also is a type of radiation; third, a radical prostatectomy (here he explained the pros and cons, effects and side effects of all these options); and the final option, do nothing. His immediate recommendation was to have a radical prostatectomy because, in his opinion, Jim was a prime candidate for this type of operation because of his age and his good health.

We wanted time to explore the alternatives, but also wanted to come to a fast conclusion. Since my nephew is an internist, oncologist, and hematologist in Chicago, Illinois, we decided we needed a second opinion. Dr. Cohen was very understanding, and, as a result, faxed all the results to him. Dr. Bob responded immediately, stating, "Uncle Jim, go for it, everything looks fine and I would recommend the same." Consequently, we made an appointment with Dr. Cohen to discuss the procedure for the operation. While sitting in the office our minds were wandering, for obvious reasons, but his office was so impressive with homemade awards and cards relating patient satisfaction that we suddenly felt more comfortable and trusting. We have been in many doctors' offices, but have never seen the likes of so much praise bestowed.

Now that Jim was at ease the conversation went something like this: Let's get this operation over with as quickly as possible. Slow down, Jim, not so fast, first we need three units of your blood (for your own protection) and the blood bank will only take one per week. Now, I have a month to think about all this. What kind of an operation is this and why three pints of blood? Dr. Cohen quickly calmed us down by telling us that the blood was just a precautionary measure and must be available if needed. The operation date was set, but in the interim Dr. Cohen explained how important it was to exercise the sphincter muscle and how often. Jim did not realize then how valuable this exercising of the sphincter muscle was until after the operation. Dr. Cohen was always such a gentleman, but he pulled no punches. He mentioned the possibility that Jim could have trouble with incontinency and/or impotency. Therefore, Jim was given a supply of iron pills. We shook hands and left. Little did Dr. Cohen know that Jim, an ex-marine, would practice his sphincter muscle almost a thousand times a day!

On our last visit to Dr. Cohen's office, he asked Jim how everything was going, always with his reassuring hand on his shoulder. Jim's quick reply was, "Get this operation over!"

Well, the big day is here, the day after St. Patrick's Day (1993), a day not easy to forget.

Now Jim is on his way to surgery and I knew what was going through his mind, especially the way he looked at me, but I kissed him and wished him luck and off he went. There were others in the waiting room, but it could have been completely empty since I was in a world of my own, not caring, just praying. Finally, which seemed like an eternity, I guess four hours or so later, Dr. Cohen said in his mild manner, "Everything went well; in fact, his operation was relatively easy and, amazingly, Jim's prostate almost jumped out at me." Well, the expression on my face told it all. My prayers were certainly answered. Then Dr. Cohen proceeded to tell me he was able to get everything out and, therefore, Jim would not need any treatments, chemotherapy or radiation. What a blessing!

Jim takes if from there:

"Dr. Cohen came in to tell me that he would release me from the hospital, and that he would have released me in two days instead of three days, except his colleagues would be upset. I thought I had the record for recovery, but today it is not unusual to be released two days after a radical prostatectomy. As Dr. Cohen left the room and went down the hallway to talk to Helen and my in-laws, I jumped out of bed, disconnected my catheter, went into the bathroom, read the directions, put on the portable catheter, got dressed, and met them in the hallway before the doctor had even left. I wore the catheter for ten days, but I was able to walk my usual two miles every day with it on. I did, however, have my own little invention that I used to make it more comfortable. I took an old pair of suspenders and cut them in half and rigged them up to the bag with velcro so I could take off the surgical rubber that was pinching my leg.

"After three days I went back to the doctor's office to have the staples removed and I felt fine. I was told to come back in another week to have the catheter removed and to bring a diaper with me. Of course I was told earlier that I possibly would have to wear diapers for a while, so naturally, I went out and bought the biggest box I could find. However, luckily, I only had to wear the one that I took to the doctor's office. Thank God for Dr. Cohen's recommendation that I practice strengthening my sphincter muscle. I never wore another diaper or had an accident. I am truly back to normal, and after seven years of physicals and occasional check-ups, I find that my PSA is .01 which reflects the wonderful care and treatment by Dr. Ross Cohen."

My brother, Steve, came from upstate New York to visit Jim and me for a week and ended up staying for three months. One evening he came to Jim and said that he was urinating blood. We immediately took him to see Dr. Cohen. He gave him an examination that included a cystoscope and told him to come to the hospital where he would scrape the walls of the bladder. This is done through the penis. After this operation he made an appointment for Steve to have a rotor rooter for his prostate. Steve returned for the operation, and just before the anesthetist put him under, Dr. Cohen told him the bad news. He had just gotten back the biopsy from the bladder and told Steve to stay in the hospital because he was going to operate on him Saturday and that it was a matter of "life and death." Dr. Cohen never operates on a Saturday, nor does the hospital provide for this. Dr. Cohen immediately made arrangements to bring in staff and have the operating room ready.

Dr. Cohen removed a malignant tumor from the wall of his bladder and kept him open until the lab examined the tumor. The lab returned with a reply that more should be removed, which he did, and then he removed a portion of Steve's bladder. The operation turned out to be a huge success. Dr. Cohen, after a couple of post-op visits, released Steve and allowed him to travel home to upstate New York. Dr. Cohen marked his stomach for radiation treatments for his prostate. Dr. Cohen also communicated with

Steve's urologist and radiologist and directed the treatment by phone and facsimile. Steve's bladder and prostate are completely healed and he has had no problems with them because of the skill and compassion of Dr. Ross Cohen.

I was introduced to this grateful survivor under unusual circumstances and he truly was given a second chance in life. General Motors was running a special clearance sale for Buick and Oldsmobiles to clear their inventory on 1999 cars and make room for their new Twentieth-century millennium cars that would soon be unveiled. It was a beautiful day and since we were invited to participate in the festivities we thought we would stop by and see what cars they had to offer. It's always nice to look, even though you are not in the market to buy. As we walked into our local Oldsmobile showroom, this pleasant-looking salesman walked over and asked if he could be of assistance. He was very courteous and went out of his way to please us. Shortly thereafter, this car caught our eye-the price was one that we could not pass up and, consequently, a sale was made. While this salesman was completing the sale, he casually asked if we had enjoyed our stay here and what we did to keep us occupied. My husband quickly said, "Play golf," and I replied that I was writing a book on a local urologist, oncologist, and surgeon. "That's most unusual, but how did this all come about?" I then mentioned how my husband's life had been saved five years ago from prostate cancer and three years ago my brother's life had been saved after coming to visit us. He had ended up being operated on for bladder and prostate cancer by this same skilled doctor. This salesman looked at both of us in amazement and said, "Was his name Dr. Cohen-I mean, Dr. Ross Cohen?" Yes, we both said quickly. He said that Dr. Ross Cohen had saved his life from kidney cancer and given him a second chance to live and smile again. After the initial shock wore off, I asked him to please give me the details.

Here is his story: "Three years ago I came home from work and when I went to the bathroom I started to urinate blood. It scared me and I quickly called my wife to make an appointment for me with our doctor. When I went to see him and after an examination, he thought there was a possibility that I might have a kidney stone. I was given medication to take in order to pass the stone. Well, two days later, I developed these awful pains from my buttocks down to my toes. The pains continued until I could not stand, walk, or sit. Back again to the doctor to get some relief. Now it seemed that my sciatic nerve was affected and I was given muscle relaxers. I felt relieved since the blood in my urine had stopped and the medication hopefully would stop the leg pains. It was difficult for me to understand how all this could have happened so suddenly, with no prior symptoms. After a few days, the muscle relaxer seemed to eliminate the leg pains-but I started urinating blood again. Well, I really was scared now, because in addition to urinating blood I had bad pains in my lower abdomen. My wife tried to calm me, but I knew something was not right. Back to the doctor now, and after a thorough examination and tests I was told to go see a urologist. I had no idea who was a good urologist. However, since I never had a real problem before, I knew I needed help fast. Fortunately, my daughter was a therapist at one of our local hospitals and said, "Dad, go see a Dr. Ross Cohen." Somehow she was able to get me an appointment quickly. After many tests, some of which I thought I would not survive, Dr. Cohen told me to dress and he would talk to me. I was very nervous, but Dr. Cohen made me feel so relaxed before he gave me the news. Very calmly, Dr. Cohen looked at both my wife and me and said, 'You have kidney cancer-but not to worry.' I remember my wife and I just stared at each other, not knowing what to say, because we were both numb from shock. Dr. Cohen said, 'You have nothing to worry about.' It was just before Christmas and certainly not a good present. After we composed ourselves, I wanted to know how quickly [treatment] could be done. Well, first, more tests had to be taken to determine the extent of the cancer. And Dr. Cohen wanted me to bank my blood, just in case it would be needed. That way, there was no chance of contamination since it was my blood.

"After all tests were completed and Dr. Cohen had explained what would be done, we shook hands and put our faith in the Lord. I gave a sigh of relief while being taken on the gurney to the oper-ating room. After six hours in surgery, Dr. Cohen came out and told my wife everything went fine. I later learned that my kidney had to be removed, my urethra and my bladder as well. However, as a result of a new technique that Dr. Cohen developed himself, my bladder was totally reconstructed and, consequently, I would not have to use a bag. Also, I did not need any treatments since Dr. Cohen stated everything was confined and had not spread. What a *miracle*. After one month I was able to return to my normal activities with very few restrictions.

"What can one say about a man like this? To be sure, Dr. Ross Cohen's name will never be forgotten. First my daughter was instrumental in getting the appointment with him, and I will forever be grateful for his 'miracle hands' that gave me that second chance to live and smile again."

One could go on recounting the many successful operations performed by Dr. Cohen. But that is why we have support groups- to hear from these grateful survivors themselves. The name Dr. Ross Cohen will forever remain in many of their minds, not only as an extremely talented, compassionate, and understanding doctor, but as a person who cares!

A SON'S MAJOR DECISION

Years earlier, when Ross Cohen was in training under his wing, Dr. Kwart spoke of his professionalism and how he was always calm and never faltered when making a decision. Like Dr. Miller, he also felt that without a doubt Ross would become a great doctor. Somehow Ross adapted himself to everything, and his concern was always the patient. Many years later, his father was the patient.

It is most unusual that a doctor would operate on one of his family-father, mother, wife or children. But, that is exactly what Ross Cohen did. Lord only knows what was going through his mind. However, when Ross learned that, indeed, his father had cancer, a decision was needed quickly. Time was of the essence, and Ross immediately consulted with his partner, Jerry Singer, and an excellent vascular surgeon friend, Dr. Jack Zeltzer.

The following are the words of Dr. Ross Cohen regarding the amazing surgery he performed on his father, Herbert Cohen.

"On April 12, 2000, my father called me at the office because he was having difficulty urinating after taking a cold pill for an upper respiratory infection. He was due to drive to New Jersey for the summer the next day, so I asked him to come to the office for me to check his urine for infection and to make sure he was emptying his bladder completely. Prior to taking the cold medicine, he had the usual prostate symptoms of a seventy-four-year-old man. My father was a perfectly healthy man with his only medical problem being mildly elevated cholesterol.

"When he arrived at the office, the urine specimen did not

show any evidence of an infection, but did show a trace amount of microscopic blood. With his history of smoking, though he quit some thirty years earlier, and since he was due to leave the next day; I decided to do a cystoscopy (a telescope examination of the bladder). The cystoscopy showed that he had several small bladder tumors, which looked like early bladder cancer. Though these tumors could have been responsible for the microscopic blood in the urine, I did an ultrasound of his kidneys and much to my amazement found that he had a 4-centimeter right kidney mass, which looked like a kidney cancer. These tumors are urologic cancers I see and treat every day, but was not anticipating having to treat one in my own father.

"I immediately sent my father to the hospital for a CT scan of the abdomen to make sure of the diagnosis and to make certain that there was no spread of these cancers. He was on aspirin, so we had to wait five days to avoid any potential for bleeding before we could operate. During this time he saw his medical physician, the anesthesiologist, and pre-registered at JFK Hospital.

"This was a difficult time for me, because not only did I just diagnose two separate cancers in my own father, but I now had to wrestle with the question of who would do the surgery. I am very fortunate to have four excellent partners, but I have the most experience and training in urologic cancer surgery. The dilemma was this: if I performed the surgery and something happened, could I live with myself? On the other hand, if someone else did the surgery and something went wrong, might I always feel guilty for not doing it myself? I discussed the dilemma with my partners, Jerry Singer, and Dr. Jack Zeltzer. Together we decided to all be in the operating room, and if I could do the surgery I would, but if I was too emotionally involved I would step aside and let Dr. Zeltzer do the operation

"On April 18, 2000, I took my father to the operating room and first removed the tumors from his bladder using the operative cystoscope. This portion of the procedure went very well, and I felt ready to go ahead with the removal of his right kidney. The rest of the surgery went exactly as planned, and the cancers were both contained, giving my father the best chance of a cure. It has been almost one year since the surgery and I am happy to report that there is no evidence of cancer and my dad is living life to the fullest. I feel incredibly grateful for that cold pill he took in early April, because if not for that we probably wouldn't have detected the cancers as early as we did."

WHEN ONE BECOMES TERMINAL

Life is so precious-and yet, for some reason, we all take it for granted. Only if you experience a serious illness, accident, or the loss of a loved one, do you finally feel the impact of life. Reality sets in and life suddenly changes dramatically. Oh yes, up until this point life is great and we feel, or think, we will all go on forever with no problems whatsoever.

During life, especially in the early years, everything seems to go rather smoothly. No need for concern because Mom and Dad most often take care of everything. Somehow, whether we know it or not, whatever problems occur, our parents are always there to help resolve them and give us the opportunity to move on more independently. As we grow older life takes many different turns. Our parents age with us, some graciously, some in health, and many needing help for various reasons. When you get to this stage, young or old, where can you turn? What can you do?

When the word "terminal" is mentioned to anyone, it frightens us. We know its implications and, unless life has become unbearable, none of us want to die, nor do we want to lose a loved one through death. The death of a loved one may also mean loss of security and of love, support, and a link with the past, companionship, and help. Facing the death of a loved one means coming to terms with our own mortality. For all these reasons, being told that someone we love is dying disturbs us profoundly. How shall we tell our loved one that unless something miraculous happens, he or she will die?

Many hospital chaplains, pastors, and doctors say, yes, tell-tell early and assure the patient of continuing support. In fact, many patients who are asked the question say, "I'd like to know. Why not give me as much time as possible to prepare?" Dr. Cohen has said that in his dealings with terminally ill people, he believes that a large percentage already know and that the dying person wants knowledge, preparation, and reassurance. Remember, doctors have feelings also-they too are human.

However, if a child is in the preliminary stages of a disease and asks, "Am I going to die?" You may answer, "All of us will die sometime. You too will die, but not today or tomorrow, or for quite a long time." But, as the child nears death and asks, you may give an honest answer: "Yes, you are dying. But don't be afraid because Mom and Dad are here with you, and all of us who love you will care for you." Adolescents can accept a prognosis that death is inevitable and convert it into an opportunity to grow.

On the other hand, trying to hide the facts or refusing to talk about them can make it very difficult for the dying person and for the survivors. But, just how do you tell? Simply, honestly, and yet tactfully. To say, "I hear you're going to die," would be too abrupt. Instead you can ask, "How sick do you think you are?" "What does the doctor say?" "Aren't you feeling better?" "You don't think you're making any progress?" Listen responsively. Your loved one may surprise you by backing off. But the next time he or she introduces the subject; he or she may be ready to talk. Match your pace with that of your loved one.

Always remember to leave open a gate of hope. Miracles do happen. Leaving open the door of hope makes it easier for the patient if he or she feels unable to cope with the diagnosis immediately. The word "hope" can have many meanings. Hope can mean remissions and many months to live. Hope can mean assurance of freedom from pain. Hope can mean looking forward to rich days with those whom we love most. Hope can mean the joyous expectation of soon being united with our Lord. Therefore, encourage hopefulness and offer courage and love when hope dims.

NEED FOR FURTHER RESEARCH
ON PROSTATE CANCER

Up until now there has been very little funding going towards research regarding prostate cancer. As stated earlier, prostate cancer was little known or even spoken about until more public figures came forward and announced that they had this "silent disease." Since then it has become a frequent news item and topic of discussion in many households throughout the country. However, unless more funding is made available for research towards this "silent disease," many Americans will possibly lose their lives unnecessarily. At the present time, retired army General H. Norman Schwarzkopf is trying to increase funding for cancer research and remove the mystery from a disease that kills thousands of Americans every year. He has campaigned to increase federal funding for cancer research since he had surgery to remove a cancerous prostate four years ago. Also Senator Robert Dole, who has appeared on nationally televised programs to speak about prostate cancer and to encourage early detection of the disease while it is still curable and which has been stressed throughout this book. This is the type of leadership needed to bring this killer disease to the attention of the public in the hope that with more awareness of its existence, more funds will be allocated for research, and more lives will be saved.

Dr. Ross Cohen has graciously accepted many speaking engagements over the years at many important functions giving information regarding urologic problems confronting both men and women today.

CURRICULUM VITAE

ROSS A. COHEN, M. D

PERSONAL INFORMATION

Office Address:	3230 Lake Worth Road
	Lake Worth, Florida 33461
Medical Specialty:	Urology (Board Certified 1992)
Marital Status:	Married, 2 children

EDUCATION

Undergraduate: George Washington University
                                     Pre Med

2121 "I" Street, N.W.   1976-1980
Washington, D. C.

Medical School: George Washington University
                                     1980-1984

School of Medicine
2300 "I" Street, N. W.
Washington, D. C.

Surgical Training: George Washington University
                                     7/1/84-6/30/86

Medical Center
901 23 rd Street, N. W.
Washington, D. C.

(Program Director: Ralph DePalma, M.D.)

Urological Training: George Washington University
7/1/86-6/30/90

Medical Center
901 23 rd Street, N. W.
Washington, D. C.
(Program Director: Harry C. Miller, M. D.)

WORK HISTORY

Urological Specialists   July 18, 1990 - present
3230 Lake Worth Road
Lake Worth, Florida 33461

PROFESSIONAL ACHIEVEMENTS AND HONORS

Alpha Omega Alpha	1984 - present
Phi Beta Kappa	1984 - present
Medical Director	Prostate Cancer Awareness Week Wellington Regional Medical Center September 1990 - present
Chief Division of Urology	John F. Kennedy Medical Center 1994 - present
Surgical Quality Leadership Committee	John F. Kennedy Medical Center February 1996 - present
Chairman Cancer Committee	Wellington Regional Medical Center 1999 - present
Vice -Chairman Quality Assurance	Wellington Regional Medical Center 1999 - present
Chairman Quality Risk	Wellington Regional

Management	Medical Center February 1994 - 1998
Cancer Committee	Wellington Regional Medical Center 1995 - 1998
Executive Committee	John F. Kennedy Medical Center 1995 - 1996
Young Urologists Committee	American Urological Association 1995 - 1996
Chairman Institutional Review Board	Wellington Regional Medical Center February 1994 - January 1995
Prostate Cancer Task Force	American Cancer Society January 1994 - February 1995
Operating Room Council	Wellington Regional Medical Center February 1994 - January 1995
Bylaws Committee	Wellington Regional Medical Center February 1994 - January 1995
Clinical Instructor	Southeastern College of Osteopathic Medicine Department of Surgery

PROFESSIONAL MEMBERSHIPS

American Urologic Association
Southeastern Section American Urologic Association
Florida Medical Society

PRESENTATIONS

Object Study Overactive Bladder - Alza Pharmaceuticals -
　　July 21, 2001
Treatment Strategies for the Hypertensive BPH patient -

July 7, 2001

The Object Story - Comparison between Detrol and Ditropan XL - June 26, 2001

South Business Report - Prostate Cancer

Treatment of the Overactive Bladder and Painful Bladder Syndrome - January 26, 2001

New Advances in the Treatment of Overactive Bladder - Detrol LA - January 24, 2001

Bladder Cancer - Diagnosis and Treatment

Painful Bladder Syndrome: Treatments of Urinary Incontinence - November 8, 2000

Effective Diagnosis and Treatment of Painful Bladder Syndrome - August 23, 2000

Surviving Prostate Cancer
Presented at Phillips Auditorium - February 2001
Good Samaritan Hospital, West Palm Beach, Florida

Neocontrol - Revolutionary New Treatment for Urinary Incontinence
Presented at John F. Kennedy Hospital, Atlantis, Florida - January 2000

Erectile Dysfunction Diagnosis and Treatment
Presented at Wellington Regional Medical Center - Prostate Cancer Support Group - October 1999

New Treatments for Urinary Incontinence, Live & Learn Series
Presented at John F. Kennedy Medical Center - February 1999
Atlantis, Florida

Urologists Play an Important Role in Women's Health
Presented at Wellington Regional Medical Center - April 1997
Wellington, Florida

Treatment Alternatives for Urinary Incontinence
Presented at Wellington Regional Medical Center Ground Rounds - March 1997 Wellington, Florida

Urinary Incontinence - Diagnosis & Treatment
Presented at John F. Kennedy Medical Center - September 1996 Lake Worth, Florida

American Cancer Society Lecture - What Every Man Should Know About Prostate Disease
Presented at the Governor's Club - March 19, 1996

What Every Man Should Know About Prostate Disease
Presented at Wellington Regional Medical Center - April
1995 & September 1996
Moderator: Prostate Cancer Symposium
Presented at Wellington Regional Medical Center - April 1995
Treatment Alternatives for Impotence
Presented at Wellington Regional Medical Center - April 1995
Update on Kidney Cancer
Presented at J.F.K. Medical Center Tumor Conference -
March 1995
Incontinence: An Overview
Presented at J.F.K. Medical Center - March 1995
I Will Manage - Part I
Presented at the Simon Foundation for Continence -
March 1995
Cures and Treatments for Incontinence
Presented at J.F.K. Medical Center
I Will Manage - Part II
Presented at the Simon Foundation for Continence -
March 1995
Update on Interstitial Cystitis
Presented at the Interstitial Cystitis Association - June 1994
Boca Raton, Florida
Urologic Complications in the PACU
Presented at the Omni Hotel for St. Mary's Hospital - 1993
West Palm Beach, Florida
Nonsurgical Management of Benign Prostatic Hypertrophy
Presented at Palm Beach Regional Hospital - 1992
Lake Worth, Florida
Nonsurgical Management of Benign Prostatic Hypertrophy
Presented at Wellington Regional Medical Center - 1992
Wellington, Florida
Nonsurgical Management of Benign Prostatic Hypertrophy
Presented at John F. Kennedy Medical Center - 1992
Atlantis, Florida
Prostate Cancer - Men and Myths
Presented at John F. Kennedy Medical Center - 1991

Atlantis, Florida

Prostate: Screening, Diagnostic and Treatment
Presented at Wellington Regional Medical Center - 1991
Wellington. Florida

Bladder Replacement Surgery/Continent Urinary Diversion
Presented at Wellington Regional Medical Center - 1990
Wellington, Florida

Nonsurgical Management of Benign Prostatic Hypertrophy
Including Balloon Dilation of the Prostate
Presented at Urology Department Grand Rounds, George
Washington University, May 1989 Washington. D. C.

Renal Scarring and Vesicoureteral Reflux in Children with
Myelodysplasia: Evaluation with Technetium - 00m
DMSA Renal Scans
Presented at the Mid-Atlantic Section of the American
Urologic Association - September 1989-Munich, Germany

Renal Scarring and Vesicoureteral Reflux in Children with
Myelodysplasia: Evaluation with Technetium - 99m
DMSA Scans
Presented at the American Academy of Pediatrics -
October 1989 - Chicago, Illinois

Renal Scarring and Vesicoureteral Reflux in Children with
Myelodysplasia: Evaluation with Technetium - 99m
DMSA Scans
Presented at the Southeastern Medical Society - November
1989
Washington, D. C.

Renal Cystic Diseases
Presented at the Pediatric Urology Grand Rounds
Childrens' Hospital National Medical Center - December
1988 - Washington. D. C.

Management of the Adrenal "Incidentaloma"
Presented at Urology Department Grand Rounds George
Washington University -
September 1987 - Washington. D. C.

Stress Prostatitis: Eminently Treatable
Presented on audio cassette by Harry C. Miller, M. D. and

Ross A. Cohen, M. D. in the Medical
Portfolio for Urologists, Vol. 6 - No. 3, 1987
Very Easy Vasectomy Reversal
Presented on audio cassette by Harry C. Miller, M. D. and
Ross A. Cohen, M. D. in the Medical
Portfolio for Urologists, Vol. 6 - No. 2, 1987

SCIENTIFIC ARTICLES

Renal Scarring and Vesicoureteral Reflux in Children with
Myelodysplasia: Evaluation with Technetium - 99m DMSA Scans
Ross A. Cohen, M. D., A. Barry Belman, M. D., Massoud
Majd, M. D., Catherine Shaer, M. D., H. Gil Rushton, M. D.

GLOSSARY

Acid Phosphatase -- An enzyme made in the prostate gland

Acute -- Reaching a crisis rapidly, having a short and sever course; sudden

Adenoma -- A benign tumor in which the cells form glandular structures

Ampulla -- A dilatation in a canal or duct

Androgens -- Masculine hormones that encourage the development of male sexual characteristics

Anesthesia -- A loss of feeling or sensation. In general anesthesia, there is loss of consciousness produced by an anesthetic agent that causes absence of pain sensation over the entire body. In the case of local anesthesia, the loss of pain sensation is localized in one part of the body. In epidural and spinal anesthesia the loss of sensation occurs from the waist down

Anti-histamine -- Any of a group of drugs used to relieve symptoms of allergies and colds. They work by neutralizing the effect of histamine, an active substance in allergic reactions

Anus -- The opening found at the end of the digestive tract

Artificial urinary sphincter -- A prosthesis designed to restore continence in an incontinent person by compressing the urethra

Aspiration -- The removal of fluids, gages, or cells by the application of suction. Aspiration needle biopsy is done by using suction through a syringe

Bacteria -- Unicellular microorganisms that may cause infection

Bacterial prostatitis -- Infection of the prostate gland caused by bacteria

Bacteriuria -- The presence of bacteria in the urine

Benign -- Nonmalignant

Benign prostate hypertrophy (BPH) -- The nonmalignant but abnormal multiplication of prostate cells in prostate tissue

Bilateral -- Having two sides

Biopsy -- A procedure whereby tissue is removed for microscopic examination to establish a precise diagnosis

Bladder -- An elastic sac that serves to store urine. The term is used to designate the urinary bladder

Bladder catheterization -- Passage of a catheter into the urinary bladder

Bladder neck contracture -- An abnormal narrowing and scarring of the bladder neck that interferes with passage of urine. Can be a complication of prostate surgery

Bladder outlet -- The first portion of the channel through which urine flows from the bladder

Bladder outlet obstruction -- Obstruction of the bladder outlet, commonly caused by prostate enlargement

Bladder spasm -- A sudden and involuntary contraction of the bladder wall, causing pain and an urge to urinate

Bone scans -- A picture of the bones obtained after the patient has been injected with a radioactive substance, which concentrates in the bones. It is particularly used to diagnose prostate cancer that has metastasized to bones

BPH -- See benign prostate hypertrophy

Cancer -- Disorderly and uncontrolled growth of abnormal cells, the natural course of which is fatal. Also called malignant tumor or malignancy

Capsule -- The structure in which something is enclosed

Castration -- In men, the removal of the testicles by surgery. Chemical castration is the suppression of male hormones by chemical means

Catheter -- A tubular, flexible instrument designed to be passed through the urethra into the bladder in order to drain urine

CAT scan -- Also known as a CT scan, or computerized axial tomography, a diagnostic technique that utilizes computers and X-rays to obtain a highly detailed image of the section of the body studied

Cervix -- Opening of the uterus

Chemotherapy -- Treatment of cancer with drugs that can interfere with the growth of cancer cells

Chlamydia -- A family of small bacterial organisms that frequently cause infections in the urethra

Chronic -- Of long duration. Chronic bacterial prostatitis in an infection of the prostate that persists over a long period of time

Coitus -- Sexual intercourse

Coitus interruptus -- Conscious withdrawal of the penis prior to ejaculation

Coitus prolongs -- Conscious postponement of ejaculation and orgasm

Congestion -- Swelling due to the presence of increased blood supply

Congestive prostatitis -- Also known as prostatodynia and prostatosis, a non-infectious form of prostatitis

Contrast medium -- A dye injected into a vein to highlight internal structures through X-rays

Creatinine -- A normal waste product filtered by the kidneys, the measurement of which in the blood is an excellent indication of kidney function

Cystoscopy -- Internal visual examination of the bladder and urethra, done with a cystoscope

Decompensated bladder -- A bladder that does not empty after voiding and loses its ability to contract

Digital rectal examination DRE (Prostate) -- An examination of the prostate by inserting a gloved, well-lubricated finger into the rectum

Diverticulum -- A pouch or sac protruding out from a hollow organ such as the bladder

Dribbling -- An involuntary loss of urine that occurs in drops, generally at the conclusion of voiding

Ejaculate -- The semen expelled to ejaculation

Ejaculatory duct -- The tubular structure through which the semen reaches the prostate urethra

Enucleation -- The removal or shelling out of a tumor from the structure that contains it, like a nut from its shell

Enzymes -- Proteins produced by living cells that help to produce chemical reactions

Epididymis -- A cordlike structure along the posterior border of the testicle that provides storage and maturation of sperm

Erection -- The enlargement and stiffening of the penis when it becomes filled with blood

Estrogen -- A general name for the female sex hormone made in the ovaries

Estrogen therapy -- The use of estrogens in the treatment of prostate cancer

External Urethral Sphincter -- Circular muscular structure which wraps around the urethra, located just below the prostate, and is responsible for urinary control

External radiation -- Radiation emitted by a radiation machine directed toward the diseased part of the body

False negative -- The erroneous result of a test when it is reported as negative, but is truly positive

False positive -- The erroneous result of a test when it is reported as positive, but is truly negative

Fertile -- Capable of conceiving and bearing children

Flow rate (urine) -- The measurement of the force and caliber of the urinary stream. If it is abnormal, it may be indicative of obstruction

Foley catheter -- A catheter that is placed in the bladder for continuous drainage and is kept in place by means of a balloon inflated within the bladder

Frequency (urinary) -- The urge to urinate very often

Genitals -- The male and female reproductive organs, internal and external

Gland -- An aggregation of cells that secrete and excrete a

substance

Grading (cancer) -- The determination of the degree of malignancy, based on microscopic evidence

Hematuria -- The presence of blood in the urine

Hesitancy -- Delayed initiation of the urinary stream

Hormonal therapy -- The treatment of cancer with hormones, or hormone manipulation

Hormone -- A chemical substance produced by an endocrine gland and carried by the bloodstream

Hyperplasia -- The nonmalignant but abnormal multiplication of cells. Also known as hypertrophy

Hypoechoic (less echogenic) -- Prostate cancer frequently appears as a hypoechoic area prostate sonogram

Impotence -- Inability to initiate or maintain an erection

Incontinence -- Inability to control the discharge of urine

Induration -- Firmness. Areas of prostate induration may be due to cancer

Indwelling catheterization -- Catheterization of the bladder with a catheter that stays in the bladder for continuous drainage

Infection -- Invasion of a body part by microorganisms, resulting in injury to tissues

Inflammation -- A condition resulting from injury, infection, or irritation. This condition is characterized by redness, heat, swelling, and pain

Internal Sphincter -- Circular, muscular fibers around the vesical neck

IVP (intravenous pyelogram) -- A series of X-ray pictures taken after a contrast material has been injected into the patient's bloodstream. This contrast material is eliminated through the kidneys and outlines the urinary tract

Lesion -- A wound, an injury, or a mass, which may be solid or cystic, benign or malignant

Lymph nodes -- Small bean-shaped masses of tissue that act as filters, filtering toxins, bacteria, and tumor cells. They are also a common site for cancer spread

Male hormones -- Substances produced by the testes and

other glands that are responsible for the male sexual char
acteristics. Testosterone is the main male hormone

Male reproductive system -- The system of the body
concerned with the production, maturation, and transport
of sperm

Malignant -- Cancerous. Having the properties of invasion
and metastasis as applied to tumors

Metastatic cancer -- Cancer that has spread from the original
organ to other parts of the body

MRI (Magnetic resonance imaging) -- A test similar to CT
scanning but in which the patient is not exposed to any
radiation and there is no known hazard. It produces
imaging of a particular body section

Neck of the bladder -- Also known as vesical neck, is the
opening of the bladder into the prostatic urethra

Needle biopsy -- Biopsy obtained through a special needle

Nocturia -- Being awakened at night by a desire to urinate

Nodule -- A small lump, generally malignant

Non-bacterial prostatitis -- Infection of the prostate gland in
the absence of any demonstrable bacterial microorganism

Occult prostatic carcinoma -- Cancer of the prostate that is
neither suspected nor diagnosed but is discovered after
prostate surgery for BPH. It is also called stage A prostate
cancer

Orchiectomy -- The surgical removal of the testes

Orgasm -- The climax of the sexual act, usually accompanied
by muscular contractions and ejaculation

Overflow incontinence -- The condition in which the bladder
remains virtually full after voiding, and urine "spills over"

Peak urinary flow rate -- The maximum rate of urinary flow
that the patient is able to generate

Penile prosthesis -- A synthetic material that is inserted into
the spongy bodies of the penis so as to make the penis
rigid enough for vaginal penetration

Potency -- The ability of a man to achieve and maintain an
erection sufficient for penetration

Prostate -- Also referred to as the prostate gland, a gland in the male that surrounds the neck of the bladder and the urethra. It secretes a fluid that forms part of the semen

Prostate secretions -- The fluid that is produced in the prostate gland

Prostatectomy -- Surgical removal of part of the prostate. The three most common types performed are transurethral, suprapubic, and retropubic. Radical prostatectomy is the removal of the entire prostate along with the seminal vesicles

Prostatic massage -- Transrectal massage of the prostate performed with the index finger, for the purpose of obtaining secretions from the prostate gland

Prostatic urethra -- The portion of the urethra that goes through the prostate gland. It begins at the bladder neck and ends at the external urethral sphincter

Prostatitis, acute, bacterial -- An acute inflammation of the prostate caused by bacterial infection

Prostatitis, chronic, bacterial -- A long-standing inflammation of the prostate gland caused by bacterial infection

Prostatitis, nonbacterial -- An inflammation of the prostate gland that is not due to bacterial infection

Pubic bone -- Bone located above the penis that forms part of the pelvis

Radiation -- The process of emitting radiant energy in the form of X-ray, light, ultraviolet, or any other electromagnetic rays from one source or center

Resection (transurethral) -- The removal of obstructive BPH prostate tissue, done through the urethra

Resectoscope -- The instrument that is used for a transurethral resection

Retention (urinary) -- The inability to void when the bladder is full. This is frequently due to obstructive BPH

Retrograde ejaculation -- The flow of semen backward into the bladder instead of forward through the penis. This phenomenon is a frequent result of prostate surgery

Retropubic -- The area behind and below the pubic bone

Retropubic prostatectomy -- Surgical removal of the prostate adenaoma. In this procedure the prostate is approached

through the lower part of the abdomen and from behind
the pubic bone

Scan -- Computerized picture of an organ or body part, such
as bones, liver, or brain

Scrotum -- The external sac of skin that contains the testicles

Secretions (prostatic) -- The fluid that is produced by the
many smaller glands within the prostate

Semen -- A thick, whitish fluid that contains spermatozoa. It
is a mixture of secretions from the prostate, seminal vesicles,
and other minor glands

Seminal vesicles -- Two sacs or pouches that are located just
behind the bladder. The secretion of the seminal vesicles
forms part of the semen

Sexual dysfunction -- A less-than-normal sexual functioning,
such as inability to obtain or maintain an erection, or
inability to ejaculate

Silent prostatism -- A condition in which prostatic obstruction
exists without symptoms, and which can lead to serious
kidney damage, if not treated

Sitz bath -- A regular or therapeutic hot bath in which the
person sits down. This can have a palliative effect on
perineal pain or discomfort

Sonogram -- A computer picture that uses ultrasound (high
frequency sound waves) to examine different organs of the
body

Spasm (bladder) -- A sudden, violent, and involuntary
contraction of the bladder wall that is generally painful
and that produces an urgent desire to urinate

Spermatozoa -- The mature male germ cell, produced by the
testicles and capable of fertilizing the ovum (female sex cell)

Sphincter (urinary) -- The ring-like muscle that a man voluntarily
contracts when he wants to shut off his urinary stream

Staging (prostate cancer) -- The process by which one can
determine whether a prostatic cancer is still confined
within the prostate gland or has spread outside of it

Sterile -- Unable to produce offspring

Stone (bladder) -- Substance formed by crystallization of

urine that remains in the bladder

Stricture (urethral) -- A scarring or narrowing within the urethra that causes symptoms of voiding difficulty similar to those of obstructive BPH. The stricture can be caused by an injury to the urethra

Suprapubic -- Referring to the area of the abdomen above the pubic bone

Suprapubic prostatectomy -- The removal of the prostate adenoma through an incision made on the skin below the navel and slightly above the pubic in the lower abdomen. In this operation the prostate is removed through an incision in the bladder

Suture -- Surgical stitches bringing together two surfaces

Testicles -- Also known as testes, the two male reproductive glands that produce sperm and male hormones. They are enclosed in the scrotum

Testosterone -- A hormone that encourages the development of male sex characteristics

Therapy -- Remedial treatment of a disease. Estrogen or hormonal therapy indicates treatment of prostate cancer by reducing the male hormone to castrate levels

Transurethral prostatectomy -- The transrethral resection of the part of the prostate, which is causing obstruction

Tumor -- Enlargement due to abnormal overgrowth of tissue. Tumors can be either benign or malignant

Uremic poisoning (uremia) -- The failure of the kidneys to eliminate excessive by-products of protein metabolism in the blood, which causes a toxic condition to develop

Ureter -- The long narrow tube through which urine passes from the kidneys into the bladder

Urethra -- The muscular tube or canal through which urine passes from the bladder to the exterior of the body. In men, seminal fluid and urine pass through the urethra

Urgency -- Acute desire to urinate, sometimes accompanied by a sensation of impending leakage

Urine -- Fluid that is excreted by the kidneys, stored in the bladder, and expelled through the urethra

Urine analysis -- The physical, chemical, and microscopic analysis and examination of the urine

Urine culture -- The incubation of urine at a specific temperature and in a specific medium so as to permit the growth and identification of microorganisms. This is the means by which an infection in the urinary tract is diagnosed

Urologist -- A physician who specializes in the medical and surgical treatment of diseases of the urinary tract in males and females and the reproductive tract in males. A urologist has had at least five years of hospital training after graduation from medical school

X-rays -- Electromagnetic vibrations of short wavelengths that can penetrate most substances of the body, thus revealing the presence of fractured bones or foreign bodies

Cancer Survivors Resource Guide

American Cancer Society, Inc. (ACS)
1599 Clifton Road, N.E.
Atlanta, GA
800/ACS-2345

American Foundation for Urological Disease (AFUD)
1128 North Charles Street
Baltimore, MD 21201
800/242-2383; 401-468-1808 (fax)

American Institute for Cancer Research (AICR)
1759 R. Street, N.W.
Washington, DC 20009
800/843-8114 (Nutrition Hotline)
202/328-7744 (Wash. DC)
202/328-7226 (fax)

Cancer Care, Inc.
1180 Avenue of the Americas
New York, NY 10036
212/302-2400
800/813-HOPE
212/719-0263 (fax)

Cancer Research Institute
681 Fifth Avenue
New York, NY 10022
212/688-7515
800/99-CANCER
212/832-9376 (fax)

ChemOCare
2 North Road, Suite A
Chester, NJ 07930
800/55-CHEMO (outside 908 area code)
908/879-4039 (outside NJ)
908/879-6518 (fax)

Coping, Living with Cancer Magazine
PO Box 682268
Franklin, TN 37068-2268
615/790-2400
615/794-1079 (fax)

International Cancer Alliance (ICA)
4853 Cordell Avenue, Suite 11
Bethesda, MD 20814
800/1-CARE-61
301/654-8684 (fax)

Mathews Foundation for Prostate Cancer Research
817 Commons Drive
Sacramento, CA 95825-6655
800/234-6284
916/927-5218 (fax)

National Cancer Institute (NCI)
Cancer Information Service
800/4-CANCER

National Cancer Survivors Day (NCSD) Foundation
PO Box 682285
Franklin, TN 37068-2285
615/794-3006
615/794-0179 (fax)

National Kidney Cancer Association
1234 Sherman Avenue, Suite 203
Evanston, IL 60202-1375
800/850-9132
847/332-2978 (fax)

National Coalition for Cancer Survivorship (NCCS)
1010 Wayne Avenue, Suite 505
Silver Spring, MD 20910
888/650-9127 (free)
301/565-9670 (fax)

National Prostate Cancer Coalition
1156-15th Street, N.W., Suite 905
Washington, DC 20005
202/463-9455
202/463-9456 (fax)

Patient Advocates for Advanced Cancer Treatments (PAACT)
1143 Parmelee N.W.
Grand Rapids, MI 49504
616/453-1477
616/453-1846 (fax)

R.A. Bloch Cancer Foundation, Inc.
The Cancer Hotline
4435 Main Street
Kansas City, MO 64111
800/433-0464
816/932-8453
816/931-7486 (fax)

US TOO International Inc.
Prostate Cancer Survivor Support Group
930 North York Road, Suite 50
Hinsdale, IL 60521-2993
800/808-7866
630/323-1002
630/323-1003 (fax)

The Chemotherapy Foundation
183 Madison Avenue, Suite 403
New York, NY 10016
212/213-9292
212/689-5164 (fax)

Vital Options TeleSupport
Cancer Network
The Group Room - Radio Talk Show
PO Box 19233
Encino, CA 91416-9233
818/508-5657
818/986-6368 (fax)

ABOUT THE AUTHOR

She was one of eight children, five boys and three girls, who was born and raised in Staten Island, New York. They were brought up as a very close-knit family, strict, but loving, and over the years moved to many parts of the country-but never too far for any of them to always keep in touch and visit. She always enjoyed and excelled in economics and finance. Upon graduation she was fortunate enough to obtain a job in the research department of a major Wall Street financial institution. Shortly thereafter, she became an institutional stockbroker dealing mainly with banks and pension funds, for over twenty five years, not only in the United States, but also in the Caribbean, Europe, and Kuwait. She will always cherish her fascinating career because of the unusual contacts she made. Although she and her husband Jim held full-time and extremely demanding jobs, they decided in 1983 to buy a lodge and country inn on a beautiful lake in upstate New York, which they ran successfully for fourteen years. They always enjoyed a challenge.

However, in 1993, her lifestyle changed dramatically. Her husband went for his yearly physical examination, and for the first time they gave him a PSA test. On the way to their new home in the south, they received a message telling Jim to call his urologist. He did so, and after a few more tests, Jim was diagnosed with prostate cancer and, shortly thereafter, had radical prostatectomy surgery. The purpose of this book is mainly to educate men in understanding the importance of detecting prostate cancer early and saving lives from this "silent disease."

Miracle Hands

by

Helen Y. Doyle

Available at your local bookstore or use this page to order.

--1-931633-43-6 - Miracle Hands - $15.25 U.S
Send to: Trident Media Inc.
              801 N. Pitt Street #123
              Alexandria, VA 22314
Toll Free # 1-877-874-6334
Please send me the items I have checked above. I am enclosing
$_____(please add #3.50 per book to cover postage and handling).
Send check, money order, or credit card:

Card #_____ Exp. date _____

Mr./Mrs./Ms._____
Address_____
City/State_____Zip_____

Please allow four to six weeks for delivery.
Prices and availability subject to change without notice.

Printed in the United States
111270LV00003B/185/A